How to Teach Continuing Medical Education

Mike Davis
Consultant in Continuing Medical Education

Kirsty Forrest
Consultant in Anaesthesia
The Leeds Teaching Hospitals NHS Trust
Yorkshire, UK

**Foreword by
Ros Roden**
ATLS® Steering Group, Chair, UK

BMJ Books

WILEY-BLACKWELL

A John Wiley & Sons, Ltd., Publication

This edition first published 2008, © 2008 by Mike Davis and Kirsty Forrest

BMJ Books is an imprint of BMJ Publishing Group Limited, used under licence by Blackwell Publishing which was acquired by John Wiley & Sons in February 2007. Blackwell's publishing programme has been merged with Wiley's global Scientific, Technical and Medical business to form Wiley-Blackwell.

Registered office: John Wiley & Sons Ltd, The Atrium, Southern Gate, Chichester, West Sussex, PO19 8SQ, United Kingdom

Editorial office: Blackwell Publishing Ltd, 9600 Garsington Road, Oxford, OX4 2DQ, United Kingdom

For details of our global editorial offices, for customer services and for information about how to apply for permission to reuse the copyright material in this book please see our website at www.wiley.com/wiley-blackwell

Library of Congress Cataloging-in-Publication Data
Davis, Mike, 1947–

How to teach continuing medical education / Mike Davis, Kirsty Forrest.
    p. ; cm.
    Includes bibliographical references.
    ISBN 978-1-4051-5398-0
    1. Medicine—Study and teaching (Continuing education) I. Forrest, Kirsty. II. Title.
    [DNLM: 1. Education, Medical, Continuing—methods. 2. Teaching—methods. W 20 D2625h 2008]
    R845.D37 2008
    610.71'1—dc22

                    2008005041

A catalogue record for this book is available from the British Library.

Set in 9.5/12 Minion by Charon Tec Ltd (A Macmillan Company), Chennai, India
www.charontec.com
Printed and bound in Singapore by Fabulous Printers Pte Ltd

1   2008

Contents

About the authors

Mike Davis was a teacher of English and Drama for eighteen years, the last twelve of which he was Head of Faculty in a large northern comprehensive school. In 1990 he moved to University of Manchester as a Research Associate in Economics Education and in 1994 became Lecturer in Adult Education in the Centre for Adult and Higher Education at that university. He led the M.Ed. programmes in Adult and Continuing Education and in Training and Development and supervised Masters and PhD students. In 2000, he moved to University of North London (now London Metropolitan University) as Senior Research Fellow in the Learning Technology Research Institute. In February 2002, he returned to the North of England to lead the BA in Education and Literacy at Edge Hill University, where he also contributed to the MA in Clinical Education. In October 2005, he became a full time freelance consultant in continuing medical education. He continues to work in higher education and holds associate posts in Edge Hill University, Lancaster University and Manchester Metropolitan University.

He has published widely and diversely (from William Blake for A level English Literature students to chapters in academic books and journals) and has attended conferences throughout the western world. He has given keynote addresses in Finland, Greece, Ireland and USA, where he was a regular visitor for six years (Department of Adult Education, University of Georgia). During this time he co-developed and taught online courses for students from American, Australian and British Universities. His Ph.D., completed in 1999, was entitled 'Learning and Teaching in Higher Education: experiences in the group'.

He first became involved in CME in 1996 as an educator with ALSG[1] working on the Generic Instructor Course (GIC). He took up a similar role with the Royal College of Surgeons (London) sponsored ATLS[2] programme. He

---

[1] Advanced Life Support Group – a Manchester based medical education charity
[2] Advanced Trauma Life Support

has directed an evaluation of the MOET[3] course and is also conducting an ongoing evaluation of the implementation and early developments of the IMPACT[4] course. He was involved in the redesign of aspects of the APLS[5] programme through the ALC-ME[6] project co-funded by ALSG and Edge Hill University. He helped design the instructor training strategies for the Level 1 RCPCH/NSPCC Recognition of child abuse course for Doctors in Training and is a member of the working party and educational consultant to the online level 2 course Child Protection In Practice, aimed at Registrars and Consultants. He has acted as educational consultant to recent developments in translating existing courses into VLE format, including:

Paediatric Life Support
Child Protection: recognition and response
Advanced Paediatric Life Support
He is currently the education advisor for the college of Emergency Medicine (UK)

Kirsty Forrest is a consultant anaesthetist at Leeds General Infirmary.

She has a masters degree in medical education (MMEd) from Sheffield University, and works in the Academic Unit of Anaesthesia, as an honorary senior lecturer at Leeds University. She organises and researches aspects of medical education, in addition to a busy clinical workload. She was awarded a prestigious three year University Teaching Fellowship (UTF) in 2006 and a Higher Education Funding Council for England (HEFCE) award to develop a local programme to improve opportunistic teaching. In 2007 she led the successful bid for a mini-project fund from the Higher Education Academy (HEA).

She is a regular faculty member on the Royal College of Anaesthetists teaching courses, and is also an educator for Advanced Trauma and Life Support (Royal College of Surgeons of England) instructor courses. She has developed several postgraduate courses and e-learning material locally, in topics as diverse as acute care and patient safety. She is co-author of the best-selling 'Essential Guide to Acute Care 2nd Ed' and 'Essential Guide to Generic Skills', and co-editor of the 'ABC of Geriatric Medicine' and 'Essential Guide to Educational Supervision'.

---

[3] Managing Obstetric and Emergency Trauma
[4] Ill Medical Patients' Acute Care and Treatment
[5] Advanced Paediatric Life Support
[6] Alternatives to lectures in continuing medical education

Foreword

"Teach these boys and girls nothing but facts. Facts alone are wanted in life... nothing else will be of any service to them."

For those who revised for A' level exams to the strains of the Carpenters, Mud and (a young) David Bowie this statement will seem all too familiar. I freely admit that I belong to this disadvantaged vintage. As a generation we laboured through medical school and many years of postgraduate education devouring yet more facts then struggling to reproduce them in a never ending procession of exams, fellowships and diplomas.

It seems ironic but appropriate that this generation of adult learners now find themselves the educators of today. We know what we have to achieve. But how to do it?! How wonderful that Mike Davis and Kirsty Forrest have produced in this gold standard publication for those of us who wish to create the most ideal of learning environments for our trainees.

This book covers everything from formal lecturing to e-learning. It explains in easy to read everyday language how to get the best out of one's own teaching abilities as well as to maximise the students' capacity to learn. The book is ideal for those who are educating and those who are learning. In particular it will provide an excellent reference point for those who teach regularly on the short life support courses. Each chapter as well as dealing with fundamentals of adult learning describes real-life teaching situations with colourful practical guidance.

As a seasoned ATLS instructor I found the section on simulated scenarios and role playing a valuable addition to my educational armoury. I would particularly encourage all ATLS instructors to read this chapter which I have no doubt will improve and consolidate their instructor skills.

As a busy clinician I discovered much of interest and practical help in the chapter on clinical teaching. I now know how I can complete an efficient business ward round whilst including some quality teaching for those accompanying me.

As a learner of the 1970s I found the book a breath of fresh air and a huge incentive to continue to develop my own competency as a teacher in this, the second half of my clinical career.

"Maintain a clear vision of your teaching outcomes. Know your audience and know your materials".

What better advice could there be?

Ros Roden
DRCOG DCH Dip IMC FRCS FCEM
ATLS® Steering Group, Chair, UK
Raven Department of Education
The Royal College of Surgeons of England
35–43 Lincoln's Inn Fields
London
WC2A 3PE

Associate Postgraduate Dean for Careers & Personal Development
The Yorkshire Deanery
Department for NHS Postgraduate Medical & Dental Education
Willow Terrace Road
University of Leeds
LEEDS
LS2 9JT

Consultant in Emergency Medicine
Regional Advisor in Emergency Medicine
Leeds Teaching Hospital Trust
Leeds

Preface

This book is intended to introduce the reader to:
- Some of the theory underpinning medical education in the postgraduate context
- A robust model for preparation and presentation of teaching material
- An exploration of a number of teaching modalities.

It is not meant to be an exclusive handbook, rather an invitation to explore some approaches that, in our experience, work with doctors at various stages of their training. As such, it is not a resource that would support studies in education at Masters or Diploma level, although we would hope that the introduction to some theory, particularly in chapter 1, might encourage you to pursue further studies.

The chapters are based on the practical experience of both authors, particularly in the preparation of instructors for Advanced Life Support and Advanced Trauma Life Support instructor courses. The invariable good fellowship and commitment of both instructors and candidates on these courses are an inspiration and a reminder that learning and teaching can be great fun. We both hope this book contributes to that.

Mike Davis
Kirsty Forrest

Acknowledgements

As quoted in *Interpersonal Computing and Technology: An Electronic Journal for the 21st Century*[1] the Australian academic, Dale Spender[2], (paraphrasing I.A. Dorner) pointed out: "as any self-respecting deconstructionist will tell you, any text is the product of other texts". I am delighted to quote this here to demonstrate the extent to which I owe the contribution of others to my thinking.

Among these are: Sue Wieteska, Chief Executive of Advanced Life Support Group who first involved me in the Generic Instructor Course in 1996; Pete Driscoll (Dean), Ruth Brown (Registrar), Kevin Mackway-Jones (Professor of Emergency Medicine) and Jacky Hanson (Chair CPD committee), Aruni Sen, Darren Kilroy and others at the College of Emergency Medicine with whom I have had challenging and interesting discussions; there are about fifteen other educators involved in resuscitation and trauma training and they have all made an impact on how I work, as have course and medical directors, notably over many years James Ferguson, John Hiscox, Ros Roden and Chris Vallis. There is a cohort of sixty or so other faculty colleagues who I have worked with on ALSG and ATLS Instructor courses and it goes without saying that these are an invaluable source of inspiration and good ideas, many of which are stolen, used and never attributed. I would like also like to mention candidates who are eager to learn and deeply appreciative of their experiences on the courses.

Kate Denning and I have worked together in a number of contexts, all of which were challenging, interesting and, in some cases, scary, if not groundbreaking.

---

[1] Davis, M. (1997), *Fragmented by technologies: a community in cyberspace* "http://www.helsinki.fi/science/optek/1997/n1/davis.txt" http://www.helsinki.fi/science/optek/1997/n1/davis.txt [accessed 4th February 2008]

[2] Spender, D. (1995). Nattering on the net. Melbourne: Spiniflex.

Kate Wieteska did the drawings, against very tight deadlines, and to her many thanks.

–Mike Davis

I would like to say thank you to Nicola Cooper for her helpful comments on the manuscript and for being the inspiration for many ideas. Also thanks to Sean Smith for helping with resources for the e learning chapter.

–Kirsty Forrest

Chapter 1 **Introduction to some theories of adult learning**

1.1 Learning outcomes

By the end of this chapter, readers will be able to:
- demonstrate familiarity with a number of theories of adult learning;
- show awareness of the contribution that it makes towards continuing medical education (CME).

1.2 Introduction

While adult learning has been described as 'an atheoretical field of practice',[1] there are some theories that are acknowledged as having a contribution to make to our understanding of the process involved in CME. These are not exclusive and there are other theories that you are directed towards in the annotated bibliography. For the purposes of this chapter, however, the focus will be on:
- experiential learning;
- constructivism;
- situated learning;
- group dynamics;
- reflective practice.

The purpose of this chapter, therefore, is to review some of the dominant methods of teaching in CME: to describe good practices; and, where appropriate, to relate these to theory. After this brief introduction to some important issues in adult learning, further chapters address each of the chosen teaching modalities, make recommendations as to their particular utility, describe good practices and suggest things to avoid. These chapters are not intended to be in any way prescriptive, but they are based on experience in education in a wide variety of educational settings. This chapter is designed

How to Teach Continuing Medical Education. By Mike Davis and Kirsty Forrest. Published 2008 by Blackwell Publishing. ISBN: 978-1-4051-5398-0

to supplement guidance from other sources and readers are recommended to look also at Mackway-Jones and Walker.[2] An annotated bibliography is also provided for those who wish to pursue issues relevant to CME further. The modalities that are of interest are:

- lectures;
- workshops and discussions;
- skills teaching;
- role play and scenarios;
- clinical teaching;
- e-learning;

and each of these is considered in turn. Before turning to these, however, this chapter considers issues related to the particular needs of the adult learner and explores some of the challenges that they bring to CME.

1.3 Adult learning

The adult learner differs from the child in a whole variety of ways, but the dominant ones relate to the extent to which adults are self-determining. This does not mean that adults are necessarily self-directed, although this should be an aspiration for them. However, it does mean that unless certain essential ingredients exist, the adult will resist the learning experience and thereby gain little or nothing from it. For the majority of learners you will meet in CME, this will not be a major issue because they will be intrinsically motivated: in other words, they will be attending the course because they want to learn as much as you want to teach. This does not absolve the course of the responsibility to ensure that appropriate and essential preconditions exist. These are often presented as a version of Maslow's Hierarchy of Needs, the most useful version of which is presented in Fig. 1.1.

This classic theory of motivation demands that much of the lower level needs have to be met before the learner can move up to the next level. In practical terms, this means that a course has to guarantee a number of conditions:

1 Adequate accommodation; regular refreshment breaks; and a working day that is tolerable.
2 A psychological corollary of 1 is that participants will need to feel safe: that they are not going to be put in a position where their ego is challenged.
3 An extension of 2 is that participants have a sense of belonging: that they are legitimate participants in the activities.
4 However, simply belonging is not enough: they have to value the group and their position in it.
5 The need to know and understand …
6 … and to value the aesthetic components of an experience.

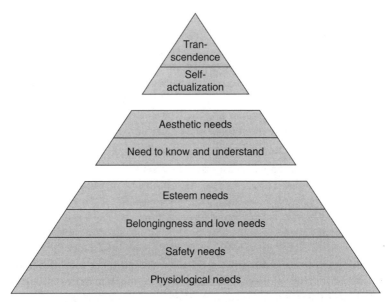

Figure 1.1 Maslow's Hierarchy of Needs. From http://chiron.valdosta.edu/whuitt/ COL/motivation/motivate.html [Accessed on 16 August 2006]

7 The state of independence and self-direction as a learner.

8 A later addition by Maslow, reflecting the desire among learners to enable other learners to achieve autonomy – this is manifested in the desire for interdependence.

Maslow's theory was based on very limited data (interviews with 140 women aged 18–28 years about their sex lives).[3] 'Maslow conducted semi-clinical interviews averaging about 15 hours with each participant. The subject of the interview included: sex drive; presence or absence of technical virginity; history of promiscuity; frequency and intensity of climax in heterosexual relations; ease of excitability; number of everyday objects regarded as sexual stimuli' and that it has never been tested empirically (i.e. how much can be left unsatisfied before moving on to the next level). This theory is widely accepted and one that makes a good deal of common sense, particularly at the lower levels. It might make some sense if you think about your own circumstances as you are reading this book. Think about:

'Am I cold, wet, uncomfortable? Am I hungry or thirsty?'

If the answer to any of the above questions is 'yes', the likelihood is that you will stop reading and satisfy the need.

'Am I psychologically comfortable? Am I receptive to some new, possibly challenging ideas?'

If the answer to any of these questions is 'no', you are unlikely to give due consideration to ideas that are new or significantly different from those you already hold.

Other levels in the hierarchy depend on learning occurring in the context of social interaction so, unless you are reading as part of a group exercise (e.g. preparation for a seminar), these do not apply to reading a book. However, I hope that it is clear that these lower level needs have to be satisfied before learning can even begin to take place.

What does it mean to be an adult learner?

It is likely that by the time you come to read this book, you will have spent quite a number of years learning: both informally in the context of parental care and family life, and more formally through school and university. As you sit and read this, remember that your understanding of it and your interpretation of the ideas are the product of many years of experience. The significance of this is that you do what you do and think what you think because you value your own behaviour and, accordingly, may be resistant to thinking and behaving differently. Try this:

Sit with your arms folded. You will notice that either your left or right hand is on top of your upper arm. Now fold them another way (i.e. reversing the dominant hand). Does this feel uncomfortable and awkward? Did you have to actively deconstruct what you need to do to achieve a (very simple) task? Many people find that this is a useful example of the challenge of doing something differently, even at a very low level in a hierarchy of learning. It could take some time and lots of repetition before you learnt the new way of folding your arms and doing it that way without thinking.

This notion of resistance to learning is explored later in this chapter. Ideas associated with taxonomies of learning are considered in Chapter 3.

What is learning?

Many doctors first come to teaching or instructing as a consequence of engagement in courses related to resuscitation in some form or train-the-trainer-type courses offered by many of the medical colleges. Many of the manuals associated with these courses describe learning as 'a relatively permanent change in behaviour brought about by planned experience'.[4] This definition has its origins in the work of Gagné, an educationalist from the behaviourist school, who argues that learners learn as a consequence of drills and repetition. There is clearly some relevance for this theory, particularly in the context of skills teaching, where there is evidence that repetition is an essential component of the learning process (see Chapter 5). However, it is an inadequate definition to describe or explain the complex changes that arise when learners' knowledge, skills and attitudes are challenged and changed.

However, change is at the centre of the process and, as we know from a wide variety of contexts, this is often resisted.

Think of the ways in which your behaviour has become routine: a journey to work, where you sit in a coffee room and, as we have explored above, how you fold your arms.

Kurt Lewin[5] argued that individuals had to go through a particular process in order to learn:

Unfreeze → change → refreeze

Unfreezing	Change		Refreezing
(1) Tension and the need for change are experienced by the person	(2) Changes are proposed by the person or group members	The person tests the proposed changes, especially those implying new behaviour and attitudes	Those new behaviours and attitudes that prove to be more productive are reinforced and internalized

Change arises from the juxtaposition of new ideas with what is already known. Lewin talked about this as a period of disequilibrium and discomfort, and learners have to be prepared to accept this. Refreezing is the process by which the learner can act on their learning and function in the world. This will be a continual process, for as long as an individual is willing, or able, to learn.

Lewin also laid the foundations for what is now known as 'the experiential learning cycle', further developed by Kolb[6] and refined as a learning styles inventory by Kolb[7] and Fry (Fig. 1.2).

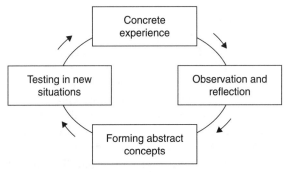

Figure 1.2 Experiential learning cycle. Reproduced from the encyclopaedia of informal education [www.infed.org]

This is a helpful source of explanation for what we do all the time: we have hundreds of experiences every day but most of them pass us by. However, if we are to learn from them, we have to be willing and able to go round the cycle, as follows.

Experience
Any event, however small.

Observation and reflection
The process of describing the event and trying to understand its significance. This stage can sometimes be captured by asking the following questions:
• what happened?
• what did it feel like?
These questions are intended to look in some detail at events and identify some of the emotional components.

Conceptualization
An attempt to generalize from the specific, by asking:
• What does it mean?
Take as an example, being late for a meeting. The focus of your observation and reflection will (inevitably) be related to that specific event (i.e. being late on that occasion) and your thinking might be: 'The next time I am due to meet my clinical director, I will set off a little earlier.' The conceptualization phase will explore being late in other contexts and the generalization would be framed in more general terms, thus: 'When I am due to meet someone, I will set off earlier than I think I need, just in case something holds me up on the way.' Therefore, this kind of thinking leads to experimentation.

Experimentation
Considering the question:
• How might I be different in the future?
Note that it is 'I' being different. It is easier to change one's own behaviour than it is to change that of others.

By going round the experiential learning cycle, a learner can capitalize on personal insight into events that are often taken for granted, but which can benefit from closer examination. Brew[8] argues that 'When we think we know, we should look again.' In the case of the vast majority of experiences, there may not be any advantage in doing this, but if behaviour seems to be working against us (e.g. in the case of being habitually late), there is some real merit in exploring experience.

Individuals have preferred styles and preferences as to where in the experiential learning cycle they are the most comfortable. These preferences are, almost by definition, context bound and can change over time. As an example, for a number of years, I taught English in high school and in order to keep lessons fresh and new for sometimes resistant learners, I put a lot of effort into experimenting with different approaches. I functioned therefore in the top left-hand quadrant, creating and providing new ways of learning. As a PhD student, I worked mainly on the bottom right-hand quadrant, where the focus was much more on reflection and conceptualization. Preferences can be identified by completing the Honey and Mumford Learning Styles Inventory.[9] This is available online for a small charge[10] and you may find it interesting to know what your preference is.

Kolb and Fry tell us that learners can be divided into:
- convergers;
- divergers;
- assimilators;
- accommodators;

and these relate to the four quarters of the experiential learning cycle (Fig. 1.3).

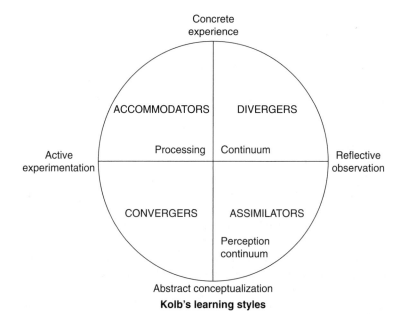

Figure 1.3 Kolb's learning styles. From http://www://www.cs.tcd.ie/crite/lpr/teaching/kolb.html [Accessed on 18 August 2006]

Characteristics of learning styles. The *convergent* learning style relies primarily on the dominant learning abilities of abstract conceptualization and active experimentation. The greatest strength of this approach lies in problem-solving, decision-making and the practical application of ideas. We have called this learning style the converger because a person with this style seems to do best in situations such as conventional intelligence tests, where there is a single correct answer or solution to a question or problem. In this learning style, knowledge is organized in such a way that through hypothetical–deductive reasoning, it can be focused on specific problems. They prefer dealing with technical tasks and problems rather than social and interpersonal issues.

The *divergent* learning style has the opposite learning strengths from convergence, emphasizing concrete experiences and reflective observation. The greatest strength of this orientation lies in imaginative ability and awareness of meaning and values. The primary adaptive ability of divergence is to view concrete experiences from many perspectives and to organize many relationships into a meaningful gestalt. The emphasis in this orientation is on adaptation rather than action. This style is called divergent because a person of this type performs better in situations that call for generation of alternative ideas and implications, such as a brainstorming idea session. Those oriented towards divergence are interested in people and tend to be imaginative and feeling-oriented.

In *assimilation,* the dominant learning abilities are abstract conceptualization and reflective observation. The greatest strength of this orientation lies in inductive reasoning and the ability to create theoretical models, in assimilating disparate observations into an integrated explanation. As in convergence, this orientation is less focused on people and more concerned with ideas and abstract concepts. Ideas are judged less in this orientation by their practical value: it is more important that the theory be logically sound and precise.

The *accommodative* learning style has the opposite strengths from assimilation, emphasizing concrete experience and active experimentation. The greatest strength of this orientation lies in doing things, in carrying out plans and tasks and getting involved in new experiences. The adaptive emphasis of this orientation is on opportunity-seeking, risk-taking and action. This style is called *accommodation* because it is best suited for those situations where one must adapt oneself to changing immediate circumstances. In situations where the theory or plans do to fit the facts, those with an accommodative style will most likely discard the plan or theory. (With the opposite learning style, assimilation, one would be more likely to discard or re-examine the facts.) People with an accommodative orientation tend to solve problems in an intuitive trial-and-error manner, relying heavily on their own analysis. Those with accommodative learning styles are at ease with people but are sometimes seen as impatient and 'pushy'.

There are a number of other learning style inventories available on the internet. Given the self-report nature of all of these, they should have little to surprise the adult learner. However, they can provide a window into something adults rarely think about and, accordingly, they can be a helpful adjunct to understanding the learners' own learning processes and those of others who they may have responsibility for.

An aside: some thoughts about the adult educator
Much of the focus of this chapter is on the learner, and rightly so. However, a major contribution is made by the people responsible for the design and presentation of the materials, and it is worth a short diversion to explore some of their characteristics.

ACTIVITY 1.1

Complete the table below:
Characteristics of teachers at various levels and the teacher–student relationship

Primary	Secondary	Higher	PG/CME
Caring	Subject specialist	Active researcher	Professionally involved

See end of chapter for responses.

Paulo Freiré, a liberal adult educator with a reforming agenda, suggested the following list of characteristics and personal qualities that teachers should possess:
- authority;
- charisma;
- consistency;
- control;
- desire for learner autonomy;
- discipline;
- expert management techniques;
- humility;
- intelligence;
- love of learning;

- love for people;
- love of teaching;
- neutrality;
- political commitment to the oppressed;
- sense of humour;
- subject expertise;
- tolerance.

He also argued that learner's needs are not always paramount in the design of the curriculum and that there are two possible agendas in any formal educational setting: Institutional agenda (IA) and Learner's agenda (LA).

The IA is dictated by the needs of society as decided by policy makers and politicians. They in turn have their own institutional and individual agendas. In this type of agenda, the individual is often seen as a function of their potential to contribute to national development; however, that is understood. The task of the formal sector is to produce a skilled workforce. An extract from a consultation document about lifetime learning reinforces this view of the aims of education, as understood by the government of the time:

> The skill levels of the workforce are vital to our national competitiveness. Rapid technological and organizational change mean that, however good initial education and training is, it must be continuously reinforced by further learning throughout working life. This must happen if skills are to remain relevant, individuals employable, and firms able to adapt and compete. (Department for Education and Employment, 1996)

In Freire's philosophy, there are types of education that are dichotomous: banking or domesticating education, and emancipatory or liberating education. The former places power only in the hands of the teacher, and the learner is seen as a passive recipient of preconstructed knowledge. He/she is prepared for a life of political alienation. The teacher is a banker of this knowledge, and makes the choices as to how, when and how much to give to the students: Teacher/banker and Teacher/learner. Characteristics of banking education include:

- The teacher teaches and the students are taught.
- The teacher knows everything and the students know nothing.
- The teacher disciplines and the students are disciplined.
- The teacher makes choices and the students comply with these choices.
- The teacher acts and the students have the illusion of acting through the acquisition of facts and skills transmitted by the teacher.

- The teacher confuses the authority of knowledge with his/her own professional authority, which s/he sets in opposition to the freedom of the students.
- The teacher is the subject of the learning process, while the students are mere objects.
- The learning process is evaluated by criteria established by the teacher.
- The teacher prepares, processes, packages and delivers knowledge and skills to the learner.

These two continua can be combined to produce a two-by-two matrix as follows:

	Institutional agenda	Learner agenda
Teacher as banker	*Conservation:* being proactive in perpetuating the status quo, and defending its superiority as a system	*Maintenance:* channelling one's energies into keeping the existing system functional
Teacher as learner	*Reform:* tinkering with minor improvements to a system in terms of equal opportunities, or improved access of teaching standards without looking deeper into causal relationships with systemic weaknesses	*Radicalism:* looking at the structural level for ways to recreate a better system on the basis of different value systems

Constructivism

In stark contrast to behaviourist theories of learning which argued, among other things, that rats could be taught how to collect rewards in mazes,[11] constructivism grew out of an alternative view of the human mind that focused on the nature of the human condition. Freidrich Hayek,[12] an early writer on constructivism, commented: 'Much that we believe to know about the external world is, in fact, knowledge about ourselves.'

Five themes encapsulate what we understand by constructivism:

1 Active agency
2 Order
3 Self
4 Social symbolic relatedness
5 Lifespan development

Active agency is in stark contrast to the passivity that is implicit in behaviourist schools of thought. Order arises from human capacity for meaning-making through patterning experience and tacit processes. The significance of self is in recognizing the nature of experience and how it is used to make sense of the world. The social symbolic relatedness arises from the social contexts within which we function. Finally, lifespan development acknowledges the relationship with what we know and new situations which we try to makes sense of over time. By virtue of the changes in life events over time, this is a dynamic phenomenon and serves as the basis of change. The significance of this theory for CME is in the extent that it contributed, along with a parallel development in social constructivism, in situated learning and communities of practice.

Situated learning

In much of formal traditional education, there is an assumption that learning is an individual effort. Learning takes place 'in the heads'[4] of individual learners and, from time to time, attempts are made to assess how much learning has taken place. This became a very powerful model that had implications for teaching at all levels of education. However, most of our informal learning takes place within a social context and is, accordingly, the consequence of negotiated meaning and understanding. Effective adult education and CME attempts to come closer to more informal methods of learning, in which learners interact with the world and try to make sense of it. When this is done in the context of other learners, it becomes 'social constructivism', whereby learners interact with one another as well as their environment. This derives in part from attempts by the Russian psychologist, Lev Vygotsky (1896–1934), to explain what happens when children learn language.

This theory was re-examined in 1991 by Lave and Wenger[13] who called it 'Situated Learning' and it is considered to have a number of characteristics which will be explored separately:
- zone of proximal development (ZPD);
- scaffolding;
- legitimate peripheral participation;
- cognitive apprenticeship;
- activity theory; and
- community of practice.

Zone of proximal development
Vygotsky[14] described ZPD as:

> The distance between the actual developmental level as determined by independent problem solving and the level of potential development as determined through problem solving under adult guidance, or in collaboration with more capable peers.

While this model refers specifically to children, it applies as much to adults entering new work or study situations: at that time, they are dependent on other members of the community for 'assistance' as they come to terms with patterns of social interaction, specific language and ways of behaving. Along with these social phenomena, they are also exposed to specific skills.

Scaffolding

Scaffolding is the operationalization of the ZPD in that it is the technique by which a full member of a community or practice provides support for the learners until they are able to manage more independently. Wells[15] identified 'Three important features that give educational scaffolding its particular character: (1) the essentially dialogic nature of the discourse in which knowledge is co-constructed; (2) the significance of the kind of activity in which knowing is embedded and (3) the role of artefacts that mediate knowing.' Responsibility for learning passes from the teacher to the learner as the learner demonstrates competence. From then on, the learner would be expected to develop full mastery and autonomy as the task becomes internalized. Scaffolding therefore can be seen as an infrastructure of information, either from prior knowledge or through teacher input, to which new material from the world can be anchored. It can involve any of the following:

- models;
- cues;
- prompts;
- hints;
- partial solutions;
- think-aloud modelling; and
- direct instruction.

It also serves to:

- provide clear direction and reduces students' confusion;
- clarify purpose;
- keep students on task;
- clarify expectations and incorporates assessment and feedback;
- point students to worthy sources; and
- reduce uncertainty, surprise and disappointment.

Legitimate peripheral participation

Lave and Wenger,[13] the originators of this phrase, wrote that learning is: 'A process of participation in communities of practice, participation that is at first legitimately peripheral but that increases gradually in engagement and complexity.' There are a number of dimensions here that need to be explored.

Legitimacy. Membership of a community is, on the one hand, by virtue of past experience and attainment, and on the other through the capacity to manifest appropriate language and behaviour. This latter may be limited in the early days as individuals come to terms with socially specific linguistic norms.

Peripherality. At first, learners do not manifest full membership of the community so they function on the edges and move, over time, towards the centre. As Hilton and Slotnick[16] write:

> This movement from periphery to centrality carries with it different 'identities'. What students do and how they relate to others (patients, nurses, doctors) is different from what house officers do, which is different from what an independent doctors does. At each stage, learners' actions and interaction provide experiences and opportunities to reflect.

Peripherality is clearly not a physical concept which is why Lave and Wenger have resisted attempts to depict it in two-dimensional space.

Participation. As is known from other contexts, there are many ways to participate. In situated learning, it is the way in which the work place enables, by virtue of legitimacy, a new member of a community to engage with its practices. Billet[17] describes this as: 'How the workplace invites and structures individuals' participation in work'. In practical terms, Eraut[18] describes this participation as:
- Group activities;
- Working alongside others;
- Tackling challenging tasks;
- Problem-solving; and
- Working with patients.

ACTIVITY 1.2

Think of your own experience as a trainee. To what extent do you recognize the above as ways in which you learnt and developed in your speciality? *See end of chapter for response.*

Cognitive apprenticeship

Apprenticeship is a helpful way of describing how learners (novices) acquire expertise under the guidance of experienced practitioners (experts). The transition from novice to expert goes through a number of stages (after Dreyfus & Dreyfus[19]):

Novice	Learns objective facts and features and rules for determining actions based on these facts and features
Advanced beginner	Starts to recognize and handle situations not covered by given facts, features and rules without quite understanding what s/he is doing
Competent	After considering the whole situation, consciously chooses an organized plan for achieving the goal
Proficient	No longer has to consciously reason through all the steps to determine a plan
Expert	Knows what to do based on mature and practiced understanding

Activity theory

Much of the development work in activity theory in relation to medicine has been undertaken at the University of Finland by Engeström,[20] who writes:

> In the model [Fig. 1.4] the subject refers to the individual or sub-group whose agency is chosen as the point of view in the analysis. The object refers to the 'raw material' or 'problem space' at which the activity is directed and which is moulded and transformed into outcomes with the help of physical and symbolic, external and internal mediating instruments, including both tools and signs. The community comprises multiple individuals and/or sub-groups who share the same general object and who construct themselves

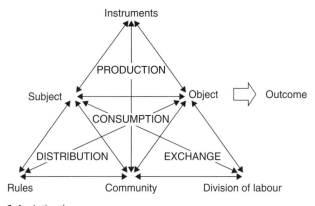

Figure 1.4   Active theory

as distinct from other communities. The division of labour refers to both the horizontal division of tasks between the members of the community and to the vertical division of power and status. Finally the rules refer to the explicit and implicit regulations, norms and conventions that constrain actions and interactions within the activity system.

This can be made more explicit by consideration of a clinical context. A patient attends an emergency department suffering from an ill-defined condition. The patient is the 'object' and the desired 'outcome' would be an accurate diagnosis and appropriate treatment, although here may be unintended outcomes arising from the treatment. 'Instruments' include assorted diagnostic tools, medical records and medical technology (X-ray, computed tomography [CT] and magentic resonance imaging [MRI] scans). The 'community' comprises other clinicians, nursing staff and other health care professionals. The 'division of labour' allocates different levels of responsibility to members of the community and the 'rules' regulate use of time (including waiting times) and measurement of outcomes.[21]

Communities of practice
In the same way that we belong to many groups, we also belong to a number of communities of practice and each has its own features:
• practices;
• routines;
• rituals;
• artefacts;
• symbols;
• conventions;
• stories; and
• histories.

These can contribute towards more global perspectives in terms of how individuals relate to, for example, their patients. In a study of the differences between doctors and nurses in their care of psychiatric patients in 1996, Robertson[22] found some similarities and differences between the two communities in respect of:
1 Beneficence:
   • utility-based;
   • virtue/relationship-based.
2 Autonomy:
   • rights-based;
   • rationality-based;

- abilities-based;
- relationship-based;

and the tensions that can exist between them.

As Robertson writes in his conclusion:

> The prime professional goals of nurses were daily care and helping patients live as normally and independently as possible; these goals were pursued through ongoing relationships whose sustenance demanded the demonstration of character virtues. Doctors' most important goals were systematic problem solving, improving organic function, and research; commitments that emphasize beneficial consequences and fit more readily into an unadulterated utilitarian mould.

This difference highlights the subtlety of community boundaries and demonstrates that while different communities subscribe to shared aspirations, their mechanisms for achieving those aims may differ dramatically. Members of communities of practice develop 'expert' abilities in manifesting the features introduced above (e.g. there are very few examples of non-clinicians managing to impersonate doctors).

ACTIVITY 1.3

By virtue of your membership of a medical community of practice, consider the following table:

Conflict between autonomy and beneficence

Within occupational groups	No of events
Doctors	
Nurses	
Between occupational groups	
Doctors advocating beneficence and nurses advocating autonomy	
Doctors advocating autonomy and nurses advocating beneficence	

Indicate 'more' or 'less' in each of the cells in the right-hand column. *See end of chapter for response.*

Group dynamics

Group dynamics as a field of study has expanded significantly, since its boundaries began to be established in the late 1940s under the guidance of Kurt Lewin and his associates.* The purpose of this section is to introduce three theories to help develop and understanding of how groups function.

Before this, however, consider the following definitions of a group from David Jacques:[23]

A group can be said to exist as more than a collection of people when it possesses the following characteristics:

- Collective perception: members are collectively conscious of their existence as a group.
- Needs: members join a group because they believe it will satisfy some needs or give them some rewards.
- Shared aims: members hold common aims or ideals which to some extent bind them together. The achievement of aims is presumably one of the rewards.
- Interdependence: members are interdependent in as much as they are affected by and respond to any event that affects any of the group's members.
- Social organization: a group can be seen as a social unit with norms, roles, statuses, power and emotional relationships.
- Interaction: members influence and respond to each other in the process of communicating, whether they are face to face or otherwise deployed. The sense of 'group' exists even when members are not collected in the same place.
- Cohesiveness: members want to remain in the group, to contribute to its well-being and aims, and to join in its activities.
- Membership: two or more people interacting for longer than a few minutes constitute a group.

Before exploring some theory, consider Fig. 1.5. Among this group of four people, how many interactions are taking place?

---

* The National Training Laboratory (NTL) was established in Bethel, Maine in 1947 and became the base for the development of the study of group dynamics. It still exists today and runs courses for managers, leaders and others interested in how learners function collectively.

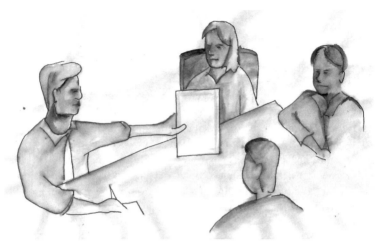

Figure 1.5   Group interactions

You might be surprised to know that there are 24 possible interactions. The answer to the questions is found by multiplying 4 × 3 × 2 × 1 usually shown as 4! If another person were to enter the group, the number of interactions would rise to 120 (5 × 4 × 3 × 2 × 1) and so on:

Number of people	Number of potential interactions
6	720
7	5040
8	40,320
9	362,880
10	3,628,800
20	2,432,902,008,176,640,000

You may think this is unlikely but it does go some way to explaining the complexity of group life.

It was this unpredictability that led Kurt Lewin and his associates to develop the science of group dynamics in the 1940s. Driven by a desire to understand how people behaved the way they did in Nazi Germany, Lewin set up experimental groups in order to observe their processes. A number of helpful theories about group life emerged from this work and the next section explores three of these. What these and other theories led to was the notion that in groups, you know what is going to happen, but you do not know what is going to happen next.[24]

Tuckman

Tuckman[25] and his colleagues argued that groups go through phases of activity:

1 *Forming:* during which time a group comes together;
2 *Storming:* when group members vie for status, leadership, etc.;
3 *Norming:* the tacit process of agreeing standards of behaviour;
4 *Performing:* when the group gets on with its set task.

This model has a degree of explanatory power and most people recognize that when (particularly) a group of strangers come together, they go through some or all of these phases.

When they first meet, they make introductions, and share some personal information and expectations of why they are where they are.

Storming often represents the biggest challenge to people's understanding as it seems to suggest high levels of disagreement and argument. However, it can manifest itself as subtle claims for status by virtue of professional role, qualifications or by virtue of charisma.

Norming is also interesting: it is a process by which codes of behaviour emerge. Accordingly, it is very unlike 'establishing the ground rules' which is often the self-appointed, and invariably futile, task of the leader of a group. The difference between rules and norms can be illustrated by this case study.

Case study. A group of postgraduate students and their two tutors are meeting for a weekend workshop designed to explore the characteristics of group behaviour in a module called 'Facilitating change in organizations'. They meet for the first time on the Friday evening from 7.30 until 9.00PM. At the end of the session, one of the facilitators reminds the group that they are to meet again at 9.00AM the next morning. When that time arrives, the two tutors and four students are there. Over the next 20 minutes or so, the remainder arrive. What follows is a long and vociferous discussion about how important it is to be on time and a rule is agreed that people are expected to be punctual. Everyone agrees to this. At the start of the next session six people are missing, and in the first session after the lunch break the two tutors are late, having been caught in traffic. Every session started without 100% attendance over the whole weekend.

One of the rules of the group was that people would be punctual. The norm, however, was that someone would be late.

Can you think of examples from your own experience where the rules suggest one behaviour and the norms another?

Norms are powerful determinants of group behaviour and it is a major responsibility of a facilitator of a group to ensure that the norms are positive and productive rather than negative and unproductive.

The final phase of Tuckman's model is performing and it is at this point that the group does the work it has come together to do.

Do you recognize this model from your professional or other experiences?

A final stage has been added to the Tuckman's model, that of 'mourning', the emotional response to the 'death' of the group. This is going to arise more often when the group has unfinished business – of the interpersonal rather than the professional (e.g. when one member of the group has never fully agreed with the group's 'choice' of leader). The popularity of websites such as Friends Reunited is an example of this sense of loss.

The most serious limitation of this model is its apparent linearity: the implication that all phases have to be visited in sequence. This is also the case with the next model.

Bennis and Shepherd

Writing somewhat earlier than Tuckman and his colleagues, Bennis and Shepherd[26] were associates and students of Kurt Lewin and were instrumental in formalizing some of the insights that has been gained through the National Training Laboratories (NTL), created in 1947 to study behaviour in groups. What Bennis and Shepherd identified was that groups would pass through two phases during their lifetime: power relations and personal relations. Each of these phases would have three sub-phases as follows:

Phase 1 – Power relations	Phase 2 – Personal relations
Dependence	Enchantment
Counterdependence	Disenchantment
Resolution	Consensual validation

Dependence. This is the state that groups find themselves in when they meet for the first time, regardless of the formality or otherwise of the setting (e.g. at the most loosely defined, people waiting to see a general practitioner in the surgery waiting room, to the more formal, people assembling for an educational event). Behaviour is cautious, and group members look for people or things to tell them what to do: behaviour can be characterized as 'flight – the fear of getting things wrong'. Behaviour is often passive and invariably obedient: 'No smoking' and 'Please turn off your mobile phone' notices are recognized as having legitimate authority. Even junior members of staff seen as being representatives of this authority can determine behaviour (e.g. 'Could you now follow me through to the teaching room', or 'The MCQ starts now'). Individuals expect to find this and are not, on the whole, uncomfortable and resentful. Indeed, if no structure were provided at the beginning of an event, there would be considerably high levels of anxiety as participants struggle to work out what is going to happen.

Counterdependence. This is often characterized by resistance to authority, often revealed as complaints about the room, the temperature, the programme and the journey to get to the venue. Members will refer to their back home status and how much important work they have given up to attend this event. This is referred to as 'fight'.

Resolution. This is the point at which the group gets on with the task: they have a sense of obligation (to authority) to complete it and there is a need to get things done. Often characterized by intense activity, this sub-phase is productive but potentially driven by external forces (e.g. status anxiety, a desire to do well, to please the instructor).

Enchantment. This is the point at which the task has been fulfilled and members of the group feel good about their achievement. They refine their outcomes and demonstrate high levels of commitment to them.

Disenchantment. This represents a standing back and an opportunity to express doubts about what a group has achieved. Individuals are uncertain about the contributions of individuals or sub-groups (think multi-agency meetings) and there is an implication (more often than not unstated) that some people did not do much to achieve the shared goal.

Consensual validation. This final sub-phase is where there is widespread recognition of the achievement of the group and the contributions (albeit different) that all members have made to this achievement.

Wilfrid Bion

Authors of the previous two models of group behaviour were sociologists, adult educators and psychologists. In comparison, Bion[27] was a psychiatrist and ex-army officer who developed his theory of group behaviour during a brief interlude in the Second World War when he was given the job of remotivating soldiers who were resistant to taking orders.

At Northfield Hospital, Middlesex, he found a group of men who seemed happy to spend their days sitting around their wards and making no effort to engage in any meaningful activity. Bion established a regime whereby all soldiers had to engage in group activity of some sort: this could be gardening, chess, keep fit. In addition, there would be a daily parade when all the men would come together to review the day. Each day, Bion would gather a small group of men and together they would wander around the various groups observing their behaviour.

What became apparent to Bion was that when they were not directly being observed, the men would waste time, lounge around, complain: anything but engage in the task. Bion concluded that groups in these circumstances were either in something he called 'basic assumption' mode or in 'sophisticated' mode.

This table may help to illustrate this more clearly:

Basic assumption (ba)	Sophisticated
Fight/flight (baF)	Work
Dependency (baD)	
Pairing (baP)	

These four modes of behaviour were considered by Bion to be exclusive: groups could not be in one mode at the same time as another mode.

Fight/flight. This is the condition in which group members either avoid the task or actively resist it by diminishing its value. Similar to dependence and counterdependence in the Bennis and Shepherd model, members' priority is to resist engaging on the task, either because it is too difficult (fear of failure) or seen as beneath them (either because of the task itself, or the environment within which the group is being asked to work.) BaF is characterized by hostility and aggression (not necessarily overt), or by avoidance of a problem or withdrawal from participation. The baF is anti-intellectual and hostile to the idea of self-study or reflection. The behaviour is invariably characterized by task avoiding, small talk, joking or attacks on the leader, the process or the room.

Dependency. The state of waiting to be told what to do: the group is unable to act without someone in authority telling them how and when they must engage with the activity. Dependency is the condition within which individuals are unwilling to act without the express instruction – either explicit or implicit – of one individual, usually possessing ascribed authority and the right and duty to lead. While a leader in baD is thought to be omnipotent and omniscient, the led are inadequate and immature.

Pairing. Somewhat more complicated, pairing is premised on the notion that the salvation for the group will arise out of the union of two of its members, regardless of gender. Other group members are not bored. They listen eagerly and attentively to what is being said. An atmosphere of hopefulness pervades the group. The group, through the pair, is living in hope of the creation of a new leader, or a new thought, or something that will bring about a new life. There is much expression of warmth, intimacy and supportiveness. It is in this ba that the group leader is not required, for within the group a new leader is going to be created, at which point, the group would shift readily to baD once more.

Work. In contrast to these ba groups is the sophisticated 'work' group, the point at which group members strive to complete their task. Bion argues that groups are very resistant to this phase and prefer to return to the relative security of ba. It is, of course, possible for the skilled facilitator to use Bion's theory in order to maintain a group in work mode. Consider the following.

ACTIVITY 1.4

A group of students are given a task to complete (e.g. to discuss strategies for implementing a new training programme in child protection), without the direct input of a facilitator. It becomes obvious to the facilitator that the group is in a state of baF. What kinds of behaviour might they be manifesting? What should he or she do? *See end of chapter for response.*

Bion's theory has, I believe, enormous explanatory power. What distinguishes it from Tuckman *et al.* and Bennis and Shepherd is that it is dynamic rather than linear, and it acknowledges some at least anecdotally accurate experiences.

Central to the success of groups, Bion believed, was the role of the facilitator, and this short extract gives a flavour of what Bion has in mind:[28]

> When I read Bion I finally had a theoretical perspective on these processes. Moreover, he said that such debacles [basic assumption behaviours] were inevitable, and they inevitably rope in the leader or facilitator. The trick is to be able to think under fire, to keep some part of your mind able to reflect on experience while having experience. If the group – or at least some of its members – can learn from experience and apply that learning to new situations, they can, just about, keep some semblance of the peace.

This is explored in more detail in Chapter 4.

Reflective practice

> We shall not cease from exploration
> And the end of all our exploring
> Will be to arrive where we started
> And know the place for the first time[29]

Or, more mundanely:

> If you think you know you should look again. Too often we close off possibilities by not looking enough.[8]

Reflection (and observation) feature in Kolb's theory of learning from experience and learning styles. However, it is the product of some earlier thinking about how we, particularly as adults, learn. Before we explore this, let us consider what it means to reflect.

ACTIVITY 1.5

Write a sentence describing what it means to reflect. *See end of chapter for response.*

Your definitions and the two dictionary ones given at the end of the chapter are probably descriptive of a process that is suggestive of fairly casual explorations of experience. However, theorists suggest it is somewhat more than this, describing the process as being about 'perplexity [and] mental difficulty',[32] 'disequilibrium'[33] and 'emotional stir-up'.[34] Dewey had a more challenging definition:[32]

> Active, persistent and careful consideration of any belief or supposed form of knowledge in the light of the grounds that support it and further conclusions to which it leads … it includes a conscious and voluntary effort to establish belief upon a firm basis of evidence and rationality.

Mezirow goes further:[35]

> A deliberate act: to develop a critique of the presuppositions on which our beliefs have been built.

Reflection on action has become a feature of medical practice in recent years but some of the ways in which it is encouraged are not necessarily likely to engage people in real reflective practice. Some examples of these are: audit, critical incident accounts and, more informally, discussions on the corridor. Rather, they will go through the appearance of reflection but are not engaging at a deep level and this will lead to replication of error rather than error correction. The target behaviour is 'reflection in action' as opposed to 'reflection on action' and this subtle alteration makes for different responses when faced with challenging situations. The use of supportive critique in many short courses is an example of an effort to encourage effective reflection. Notwithstanding this, there are some challenges.

Barriers to reflection
- Presuppositions about what is and what is not possible for us to do.
- Not being in touch with one's own assumptions and what one is able to do.
- Past negative experiences.
- Expectations of others: society, peer group, figures of authority and family.
- Threats to the self, one's world view or to ways of behaving.
- Lack of self-awareness of one's place in the world.
- Inadequate preparation.
- Hostile or impoverished environments.
- Lack of opportunity to step aside from tasks.
- Lack of time.
- External pressures or demands.
- Lack of support from others.
- Lack of skills: in noticing, intervening.

- Intent that is unclear or unfocused.
- Established patterns of thought or behaviour.
- Inability to conceive of the possibility of learning from experience: 'this is not learning', 'this is not possible'.
- Stereotypes of how we learn.
- Obstructive feelings: lack of confidence or self-esteem, fear of failure or the response of others, unexpressed grief about lost opportunities.[36]

Reflection is not an easy option and it may involve challenging some comfort zones if learners are going to gain full advantage from their experiences.

Conclusions

In this chapter we have explored some important theories of adult learning and how these relate to CME. In the following chapter, we explore the extent to which these can be realized in practice.

References

1 Knowles M. *The Adult Learner: A Neglected Species* (4th edn). 1990. Gulf Publishing, Houston and London.

2 Mackway-Jones K, Walker M. *The Pocket Guide to Teaching for Medical Instructors (Advanced Life Support Group).* 1999. BMJ, London. [A new edition of this book will be available in 2008. Bullock I, Davis M, Lockie A, Mackway-Jones K (eds.). *Pocket Guide to the Principles of Education* (2nd edn). Blackwell, Oxford.]

3 Alimo-Metcalfe B. Maslow: A different view. *The Psychologist* 2001;**14** Part 4 http://www.thepsychologist.org.uk/archive/archive_home.cfm/volumeID_14-editionID_14-editionID_55-ArticleID_195-getfile_getPDF/thepsychologist/paininbum.pdf (accessed 3 February 2008)

4 Gagné R. *The Conditions of Learning* (4th edn). 1985. Holt, Rinehart & Winston, New York.

5 Lewin K. *Field Theory in Social Science.* 1951. Harper & Row, New York.

6 Kolb D. *Experiential Learning: Experience as the Source of Learning and Development.* 1984. Prentice-Hall, Englewood Cliffs, NJ.

7 Kolb D. https://www.cs.tcd.ie/crite/lpr/teaching/kolb.html [accessed on 16 August 2006]

8 Brew A. Unlearning through experience. In Boud D, Cohen R, Walker D. (eds.) *Using Experience for Learning.* 1993. SRHE/Open University Press, Buckingham.

9 Honey P, Mumford A. http://www.campaign-for-learning.org.uk/about yourlearning/whatlearning.htm [accessed on 16 August 2006]

10 http://www.peterhoney.com/LS80/index [accessed on 26 August 2006]

11 Watson J, Rayner R. Conditioned emotional reactions. *Journal of Experimental Psychology* 1920;**3**:1–14.

12 Hayek F. *The Sensory Order*. 1952. University of Chicago Press, Chicago.

13 Lave J, Wenger E. *Situated Learning: Legitimate Peripheral Participation*. 1991. University of Cambridge Press, Cambridge.

14 Vygotsky L. *Mind and Society: The Development of Higher Mental Processes*. 1978. Harvard University Press, Cambridge, MA.

15 Wells G. *Dialogic Inquiry: Towards a Sociocultural Practice and Theory of Education*. 1999. Cambridge University Press, New York.

16 Hilton S, Slotnick H. Proto-professionalism: How professionalisation occurs across the continuum of medical education. *Medical Education* 2005;**39**:58–65.

17 Billett S. Toward a workplace pedagogy: Guidance, participation and engagement. *Adult Education Quarterly* 2002;**53**:27–43.

18 Eraut M. Informal learning in the workplace. *Studies in Continuing Education* 2004;**26**:247–273.

19 Dreyfus H, Dreyfus, S. (1986), *Mind over Machine: The Power of Human Intuition and Expertise in the Era of the Computer*. Basil Blackwell, Oxford.

20 Engeström Y. *Learning by Expanding: An Activity–Theoretical Approach to Developmental Research*. 1987. Orienta-Konsultit, Helsinki.

21 http://www.edu.helsinki.fi/activity/pages/chatanddwr/activitysystem/ [accessed on 2 May 2007]

22 Robertson D. Ethical theory, ethnography, and differences between doctors and nurses in approaches to patient care. *Journal of Medical Ethics* 1996;**22**:292–301.

23 Jacques D. *Learning in Groups*. 2000. Kogan Page, London.

24 Davis M. Reflections of a co-trainer. *Groupvine* 1993;**1**:13–14.

25 Tuckman B. Developmental sequence in small groups *Psychological Bulletin* 1965;**63**:384–399.

26 Bennis W, Shepherd H. A theory of group development. *Human Relations* 1956;**9**:415–437.

27 Bion W. *Experiences in Groups*. 1961. Tavistock Press, London.

28 Young R. Bion and experiences in groups. 2005 http://human-nature.com/rmyoung/papers/pap148h.html [accessed on 21 August 2006]

29 Eliot TS. Little Gidding. *The Four Quartets*. 1943. Faber, London.

30 *Collins English Dictionary*. 1998, 9th edition.

31 *Webster's International Dictionary*. 1993, 3rd edn.

32 Dewey J. *How We Think*. 1933. DC Heath, Boston, MA.

33 Blumberg A, Golembiewski R. *Learning and Change in Groups*. 1976. Penguin, Harmondsorth.

34 Lewin K. Frontiers in group dynamics: Concept, method and reality in social science; social equalibria and social change. *Human Relations* 1947;**1**:2–38.

35 Mezirow J. How critical reflection triggers transformative learning. In *Fostering Critical Reflection in Adulthood* Mezirow J *et al.* (eds.) 1990. Jossey-Bass, San Francisco, CA.

36 Boud D, Cohen R, Walker D. *Reflection: Turning Experience into Learning*. 1985. Kogan Page, London: p. 79.

Responses to Activities

Activity 1.1

Characteristics of teachers at various levels and the teacher–student relationship

Primary	Secondary	Higher	PG/CME
Caring	Subject specialist	Active researcher	Located in community of practice
Fostering social norms	Fostering social norms	Inducting students into the academic community	Maintaining standards of professional practice
Formative	Formative	Lecturer	Facilitator
Unequal power relations	Unequal power relations	Hierarchical	Assessor
Child-centred	Subject-centred	Constrained by institutional demands	Mentor
Somewhat constrained by external forces (assessment at 5, 7 & 11)	Constrained by institutional demands	Supervisor	
	Constrained by external forces (assessment at 14, 16, 17 & 18)	Examiner	

Activity 1.2

As a trainee in anaesthesia, the first few weeks consist of being on the periphery. You do not have the knowledge or skills to perform any of the skilled tasks. However, you were part of the group, expected to visit patients and observe the process of anaesthesia. It was a whole new world of machines and words that I had not heard of before, but gradually you were allowed more responsibility, allowed to perform parts of the performance but not all at once. It had a community feel from the start, it was all about team work and I suppose working in a technical service specialty really emphasizes that.

The way I really remember the progression of participation through training is thinking about emergency abdominal aortic aneurysm repairs. These are true emergencies that anaesthetists are involved in and usually there is more than one anaesthetist present.

The first one I saw was as an SHO – all I remember was standing in corner thinking that looks like a lot of blood, watching the other anaesthetists running around and wondering how did they know what to do. The second time I had the important job of recording the vital signs, what was done to the patient, counting blood bags and syringes, filling in forms and answering phone calls. The third time I performed the skills like canulation, line insertion and squeezing the blood bags.

When I was a registrar, I would direct the SHO what to do, call the consultant (if not present), inform the surgeon of blood loss, order more blood and products, arrange an intensive care bed and feel like I was running the show. As a consultant I oversee the registrar and, depending on their seniority and experience and patient factors, may actually become the scribe again.

Activity 1.3

Conflict between autonomy and beneficence	
Within occupational groups	*No of events*
Doctors	15
Nurses	24
Between occupational groups	
Doctors advocating beneficence and nurses advocating autonomy	8
Doctors advocating autonomy and nurses advocating beneficence	1

Activity 1.4

The group will be engaging in small talk, will be drawing on back-home status to justify their opinions, they will criticize the task or make negative comments about the facilitator and will talk about how much more important it would be for them to be back at work. The extent to which this continues will be determined by their levels of motivation: if they have been 'pressed' to attend, this may be significant.

The facilitator should put the group in dependency mode: 'OK, let us think about the progress so far ...' and then restate the requirements of the task. While possibly continuing to manifest signs of baF, the group may have sufficient motivation to move into work.

Activity 1.5

Definitions range from the general: 'Careful or long consideration or thought'[30] to somewhat more specific: 'Mental consideration of some subject matter, idea or purpose, often with a view to understanding or accepting it, or seeing it in its right relations.'[31]

Chapter 2 **Teaching design and presentation**

In the previous chapter, we explored some of the theories that help us to understand what happens among learners when they engage in formal education. In this chapter, we look at the structure of a teaching event: what it means to prepare and carry out a session by maximizing resources (including those of the facilitator) and minimizing distracting influences.

2.1 Learning outcomes

By the end of this chapter, you will be able to:
• recognize and evaluate a learning event; and
• recognize a robust structure and its capability of being applied to any setting, from a small workshop to a presentation in a large conference.

Regardless of the teaching modality, an absolutely essential component of a session is preparation and this is the focus of the next section.

2.2 Preparation

A good rule of thumb is that you need at least as much time to prepare as you do to deliver a session. This depends on the novelty of the material: if it is completely new, you may be spending a considerable time working out what you are going to do and how.

People will develop their own strategies for preparation, but it may involve a number of steps:
• *Identifying source material:* this could be existing literature or interpretations of new data.
• *Sourcing appropriate materials:* URLs, clinical slides, audio or video clips and algorithms.

How to Teach Continuing Medical Education. By Mike Davis and Kirsty Forrest. Published 2008 by Blackwell Publishing. ISBN: 978-1-4051-5398-0

- *Planning the session:* designing the session. This is more straightforward for a lecture, but can be quite complex for more interactive sessions.
- *Preparing audiovisual resources:* this could involve creating a powerpoint presentation (see below), developing other materials, photocopying resources.

ACTIVITY 2.1

You have been asked to run an interactive session lasting 1 hour at a short in-house training event. What do you need to consider:

  a) 1 week before;
  b) 1 day before;
  c) 1 hour before the session.

What do you do at the last minute?

Many of these may be self-evident but the ones that are not, are those that can catch you out. *See end of chapter for response.*

2.3 Preparation and initiation

Set, to be explored more fully later in the chapter, can be described as 'a psychological frame of mind in which learners are prepared to learn'[1] and it comprises issues related to the physical space in which learning takes place, and the cognitive and affective climate that is created by the facilitator. In the first instance, however, let us focus on environment.

Environment

While it is true to say that facilitators do not always have control of the classroom space for their sessions, they can minimize negative impact by some careful preparation and attention to organizational detail. As far as possible, you should think about light, heat and equipment and this invariably means visiting the room in advance of the session. Light levels are particularly important if you are using a data projector – overhead projectors are more forgiving. Temperature should be controlled by opening windows or adjusting the air conditioning, before and between sessions. However, be aware of the impact of external noise if windows are to be left open. Do not compete with loud internal noise (e.g. fans, heaters, air conditioning). Any equipment you are planning to use in your session needs to be checked for: (a) effective working; and (b) familiarity. Data projectors and computers vary and older ones may not have accessible USB ports for memory sticks; newer ones may not have disc drives.

During this time, it is possible to adjust classroom furniture in order to create the most appropriate classroom space for the teaching modality to be employed. Invariably, rooms are left set up for lectures as described in a later chapter. If you are planning another modality, you may have to take responsibility for moving furniture. Attention to classroom layout is paid in later chapters.

Set

This is the initiation stage of a teaching situation during which time you subtly establish a number of preconditions for effective participation in the session. You should be in the room a couple of minutes before your session is due to start. If you are following another person, all you have to do is walk to the front of the room in front of your audience. If you are the first (e.g. after a break), you can make a quiet entrance and wait for the group to assemble.

Timekeeping

Invariably, when a course is being prepared, the organiser will send out a programme indicating where and when events are to take place. It is important that the course as a whole adheres to this timetable: remember that participants may have had to make arrangements (e.g. for child care) so finishing on time is important. Each session leader contributes to the overall achievement of this implied contract so it is important not to exceed the time you have been given. In some settings (e.g. conferences), time keeping is left to a chairperson and is often rigidly imposed. It is important therefore that you are capable of developing your session to fit the time available.

ACTIVITY 2.2

Consider this case study:

Twenty four learners have come together for a 3-day course on training the trainer. The first 15 minutes of the day, after registration and coffee, is spent in mentor groups where learners and facilitators spend time getting to know one another and establishing arrangements for support and guidance throughout the 3 days. At 9.15 AM, everyone gathers in the plenary room for the opening session to be led by the course director. He is not there and does not arrive until 9.30 AM, after which his 15-minute session overruns by 10 minutes.

What norms do you think will have been established by this behaviour? You may need to refresh your memory about norms in Chapter 1. *See end of chapter for response.*

ACTIVITY 2.3

What do you do when you realise at the time you are due to start that there are participants still missing? *See end of chapter for response.*

When you are ready to start, introduce yourself briefly and lay claim to your expertise in the area. This is not immodest and it does add to your credibility. For example, 'My name is Jack Ripper and I am a consultant in Emergency Medicine and I am going to talk to you today about something I find particularly interesting because of its increasing incidence on the streets of our cities: stab wounds.' However, your ultimate credibility arises from your ability to run your session effectively, giving your learners valuable information and insight.

It is always useful to confirm the session title and to indicate its purpose, perhaps in terms of 'learning outcomes' – statements of what the learners can be expected to have learnt by the end of the session. This can serve to give the candidates a sense of the structure of the session, the order they are likely to engage in the subject matter and an indication of its place in the course as a whole. It is not necessary to assert importance for the session: this should be assumed, but it can be useful to suggest *why* it is important (e.g. in a demonstration of the log roll, you could emphasize the importance of examining for occult injuries).

You may wish to say what the learners' roles are to be so, for example, they are not taken by surprise if you ask them questions or you ask them to engage in group activity as part of the session.

Dialogue
This is the heart of the session when you deal with the substantive issues. Your role in this phase is to enable students to develop and refine their understanding. You can do this in a number of ways:
- *Explaining:* essentially a passive role for the learner, but can be valuable.
- *Exploring:* posing problems and examining them from a number of perspectives. You may want to engage the learners in this process.
- *Critiquing:* offering a challenge to the interpretation.
- *Questioning:* see the variety of question types below.
- *Summarizing:* not closure (see below) but short summaries to remind learners what they have covered so far and where you are going next.
- *Responding:* to questions or non-verbal behaviour that demonstrates doubt or uncertainty.

There will be more about dialogue in each of the following chapters as the dialogue can differ in each modality.

Closure

As we have already discussed, time is the key variable that tells you that you have to move towards closure. You need to leave up to 5 minutes at the end of a session to go through the following sequence:

- 'Are there any questions?'
- Be prepared to wait about 10 seconds (count: one elephant, two elephants ...).
- When you are asked a question, it may be useful to repeat it, either verbatim or by paraphrasing.

ACTIVITY 2.4

Why might you consider this to be valuable? *See end of chapter for response.*

Answer all questions or, if time begins to press, arrange to meet questioners during a break. Actively seek them out although they may not actually want to know the answer. Motives for asking questions are varied: in the worst case, someone is asking in order to make them appear intelligent, insightful, in touch with new research. Not only may they be trying to impress you, they could be trying to impress their fellow candidates and once the audience has gone, they lose that opportunity.

If you do not know the answer, say so. There is nothing wrong with saying that you will have to check something. However, making something up, or being vague or answering a different question will undermine your credibility. If this situation arises, tell the audience that you will find out from a colleague. It is then important then that you do so and communicate the answer to the questioner. If it is a particularly important issue, you may want to give the answer at the next plenary session.

The final element is the opportunity to have the last word: the summary. 'In summary, what we have done in this session is (revisit the learning outcomes and deliver the take-home message).'

Summarize what the candidates have learnt, including any important issues raised during questions. This should then be followed by termination. 'You should now move on to the next session/coffee/etc.'

Do not be drawn into questions at this time. Questioners are usually trying to demonstrate their superior insights and they are pursuing personal agendas at the expense of the group as a whole. Talk to them over coffee. It may be that they will not want to pursue their question as they no longer have an audience.

Some thoughts on asking questions

Questions are an important component in any teaching modality. At the most basic, they can check knowledge ('What is the normal range for the pH of the blood?') to the ability to evaluate complex data from multiple sources.

Appropriate questions are intended to reflect the levels of knowledge that candidates might reasonably expect to have:

- *knowing:* to identify; name; describe;
- *understanding:* to compare; distinguish; show;
- *applying/analysing:* to specify; demonstrate; hypothesize;
- *synthesizing:* to create; speculate; design;
- *evaluating:* to assess contribution of differing perspectives.

This hierarchy is drawn from the work of Bloom and his associates,[2] who identified levels of achievement in terms of knowledge, skills and affect. We will be looking more closely at the implications of these for the various teaching modalities in later chapters but, as an introduction, consider these questions:

- In what year was the Battle of Hastings?
- In what ways was that battle different from the Battle of Britain, for example?
- What were William's motives in launching his campaign?
- How long was it before William was able to establish a Norman hegemony in England? What particular strategies did he employ?
- What was the impact on the development of the English language as a consequence of the Norman invasion?

Or, in a medical example:

- What are the causes of shock in a trauma patient?
- In what way do they cause hypotension?
- How can you differentiate between the different types of shock?
- What are the strategies for treating shock?
- Which fluid would you use for resuscitation?
- What do you think about low volume resuscitation?

You might find you know the answer to the lower level questions but as you travel up the hierarchy questions get less easy to answer and depend on considerably more than facts. Unlike Gradgrind, the medical educator must think beyond the notion that facts alone are important:[3]

> What I want is, Facts. Teach these boys and girls nothing but Facts. Facts alone are wanted in life. Plant nothing else, and root out

everything else. You can only form the minds of reasoning animals upon Facts: nothing else will ever be of any service to them. This is the principle on which I bring up my own children, and this is the principle on which I bring up these children. Stick to Facts, sir!

References

1 American College of Surgeons Committee on Trauma. *ATLS Student Course Manual* (7th edn). 2004. American College of Surgeons, Chicago.
2 Bloom B. *Taxonomy of Educational Objectives.* 1984. Alleyn & Bacon, Boston, MA.
3 Dickens C. *Hard Times.* 1995. Penguin, Harmondworth.

Responses to Activities

Activity 2.1

One week before the event
Prepare – anything from gathering notes to initiating literature review.

Decide on the use of audiovisual aids and prepare the materials. In most cases, this will involve a PowerPoint presentation.

Be in contact with the local organizer to ensure what to expect in terms of the environment in its broadest sense. Questions to ask include:

- How big is the room?
- Is it warm/cold?
- Is there air conditioning?
- Are there PowerPoint and projection facilities?
- Can the PC accept a memory stick/CD?
- Is their an Internet connection in the room?
- Is the furniture fixed?
- How big an audience can I expect?
- Who are they (e.g. consultants, medical students)?

Practice your session. This does not mean doing it in front of a mirror (or significant other) but it does mean that you should 'walk through' the session, reminding yourself of what are planning to do and your thinking behind it. Identify significant landmarks to assist in your timing.

One day before the session
- Check your materials.
- Save presentation to flash drive and back up to other media.
- e-mail it to yourself.
- Contact the organizer to check for any change of plan.

One hour before the event

Check the room and confirm that the computer will accept your data. Load it onto the desktop (this will maximize speed and handling, particularly if you have animations, audiovideo streams from CD/DVD or Internet links). Check water supplies – even the most experienced facilitators can suffer from a dry mouth. If you are going to use a flip chart or a white board, check that the markers are of the right type and that they work. Make sure you have enough flip chart pages for the session. Prepare flip charts if necessary. You can do this by writing on the flip chart in pencil using small letters, e.g.

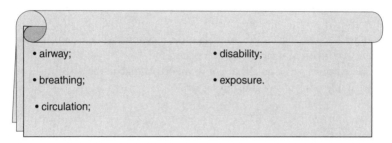

- airway;
- breathing;
- circulation;
- disability;
- exposure.

You will be able to see it but even those closest to the flip chart will not. This is particularly useful if you have a complex diagram or algorithm.

In the final minute, you should focus on what is to follow. Make sure that you have everything you need.

Activity 2.2

The main norm for the group to emerge from this session was that it was acceptable to start late. Every single session over a 3-day period overran. The consequences were longer days and significant loss of time for coffee and lunch breaks. The knock-on effect of the former can be significant for learners who may have made arrangements for times in the day that were not programmed (e.g. child care). The loss of refreshment breaks in the course results in a failure to provide adequately for physiological needs.

Activity 2.3

This depends on a number of circumstances, depending on where your session is in the programme.

If yours is the first session, in consultation with the programme organizer, you may be able to announce a short delay to allow for travel, parking problems, etc. However, this should not be significant – no more than 15 minutes. The course programme is, in my view, a contract that you should try to honour and late starts/finishes can cause disruption and make candidates anxious and/or irritated. The lost time can usually be made up, either by shortening the session or by cutting into coffee or lunch breaks later in the day.

If your session follows a coffee break, allow no more than 2 minutes before you start. It may be that otherwise you would be inconveniencing (say) 20 people at the expense of one or two. When latecomers arrive, however, acknowledge their presence and quickly let them know where you are up to.

Activity 2.4

Repeating or paraphrasing provides a number of advantages:
- It gives you some thinking time.
- It gives the learners some thinking time: they too will be formulating an answer as part of their internal dialogue.
- Some people speak quietly and it is important that all the audience know what question you are going to answer.

Chapter 3 **The lecture**

The purpose of this chapter is to explore the contribution of the lecture to learning.

The learning outcomes are to:
- identify strengths and weaknesses of the lecture;
- describe the characteristics of the lecture;
- describe how to ask questions in a variety of ways;
- describe how to ask questions at a variety of levels.

ACTIVITY 3.1

Think about the best lecture you have ever heard. List its qualities. Compare your thoughts with those shown at the end of the chapter. *See end of chapter for response.*

The question that this inevitably leads to is 'What is the purpose of a lecture?'

3.1 Advantages of the lecture

Lectures play an important part in much of continuing medical education (CME). It is clear therefore that they are considered to have some advantages over other ways of teaching:

1 *Economic:* one lecturer, many students. It is not uncommon in undergraduate education to find hundreds of students in large lecture theatres; televized lectures can reach millions of people. However, most CME is rarely presented to these numbers and you are far more likely to have 20–30 in your audience.

2 *Disseminate information:* lectures often are used to supplement the release of new or updated course manuals or to introduce new protocols

How to Teach Continuing Medical Education. By Mike Davis and Kirsty Forrest. Published 2008 by Blackwell Publishing. ISBN: 978-1-4051-5398-0

(e.g. in resuscitation training). They may report findings of clinical or other studies; they may introduce new procedures. Invariably, verbal presentations are supplemented by written information, where learners can revisit the issues in their own time.

3 *Stimulate learner interest:* to be followed up by any number of additional activities – reading, (Internet) research, skills learning, simulations, etc.

4 *Reduce ambiguity* (theoretically, at least): the audience hear the same message. However, there is evidence to suggest that not all members of an audience hear the same message. Indeed, some learners are not listening to the message at all. The radical adult educator Paulo Freire (see Chapter 1) was deeply critical of the lecture as a modality for a number of reasons, some pragmatic and others more conceptual. At the most mundane, he argued that students in a lecture would engage in a range of distracting activities: reading, talking, sleeping and writing shopping lists. However, his more profound criticisms were about the design of the educational experience that had the lecture at its heart:[1]

> Currently in education, there is excessive use of lecturing and memorization, with little analysis of the importance of what is being memorized. For example, 1945 marks the end of the Second World War, but we do not know how that affected our lives or how it continues to affect the daily relationships we establish. We have simply memorized and retained the date. Freire describes this situation as one in which the students are seen as containers into which knowledge can be deposited. The teacher is the depositor and the knowledge is that which is deposited on a daily basis. This bank concept of education attempts to transform the minds of individuals so that they will adapt better to actual situations and be dominated by them with greater ease. The more passive people are, the more they will adapt, the more their creativity will diminish and their naiveté increase, which creates the conditions necessary for the oppressors to emerge as generous benefactors.

3.2 Limitations of a lecture

Lectures have other limitations:

1 *Inadequate for skills teaching:* skills require a different structure (see Chapter 5), fewer numbers and close audience proximity.

2 *Not necessarily good for abstract or complex issues:* its ethereal nature do not lend themselves to deep thought, complex sentence structures or reflection.

3 *Hard to integrate the content of a lecture with other teaching sessions:* reference can be made to other sessions, but detailed exploration of the inter-relationships are more complex.

4 *Make significant demands on the attention span of an audience:* research suggests that for most people they can concentrate for around 40 minutes before there is significant decay in their ability to 'hear' what is being said. A classic study[2] published in 1978 argued that from a high at 10–15 minutes, concentration declines rapidly. This does not mean that lectures need to be limited to 15 minutes; rather it suggests that other activities are built into the session. This is explored in more detail below.

3.3 Structure

The structure of a lecture, as with other teaching modalities, needs to follow that already introduced in Chapter 2, but with some particular features that you need to pay attention to.

Set (including environment)

Environment

The layout for a lecture is what you tend to find when you walk into a classroom in any university or postgraduate centre: rows of chairs or fixed furniture pointing towards a screen of some kind (Fig. 3.1). There may or may not be a lectern. Almost invariably, there will be an assortment of visual aids, ranging from computers and data projectors through to blackboards

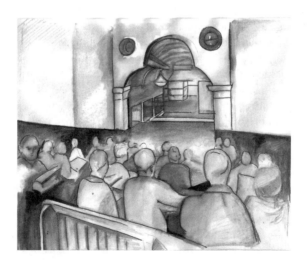

Figure 3.1 The traditional lecture theatre

or whiteboards. In some settings, you may also find interactive whiteboards or similar, more advanced technology.

ACTIVITY 3.2

What do you consider to be the advantages and disadvantages of an assortment of audiovisual aids?
   Complete the following table:

A/V aid	Pros	Cons
Black/whiteboard		
Overhead projector		
Flip chart		
35 mm slide projector		
Video/DVD player		
Computer + data projector		
Interactive whiteboard		

See end of chapter for response.

It might be argued that the more sophisticated systems are, the more likely they are to go wrong. My experience, however, is that if you plan carefully, arrive well in advance of your session (in order to check everything), have back-up equipment and materials (e.g. your own laptop; two versions of your file on a data stick. I often email a presentation to myself) and a fallback strategy (overhead transparencies slides, if absolutely desperate), you should be able to deliver your lecture without too much in the environment making your life difficult.

As you will recall from Chapter 1, physiological needs have to be met before learning can take place. However, in most lecture environments, heat and light almost always demand compromises: a room may be well ventilated at the beginning of a session, but warm and stuffy by the end. Open windows or air conditioning may be noisy. It is important to plan to change the environment if and when the opportunity presents itself. For example, if you set a group task during your lecture, you could open windows or turn the air conditioning on until you are ready to speak again to the whole group.

Layout is much more in your control, if only as to where your audience sits. If, for example, you have 20 students in a large lecture theatre, ask them to come and sit close to the front, in the middle. This gives you less of a problem of projection, interactivity and eye contact. For some reason, students inevitably drift towards the back of a space and are especially reluctant to sit on the front row. However, a study in the USA[3] discovered that students who sit near the front are more attentive and get higher grades, despite their initial preference for where they sit.

Ensure that the screen is visible from all angles, paying particular attention to extremes (left or right) and to the existence of any obstacles to a view of you, or the screen. If you are using a data projector, ensure that it is readily accessible to enable you to move through the slides. If there is a remote control, make sure you know how it works. If you plan to use a flip chart or whiteboard, make sure that the marker pens work and that there are sufficient clean pages for you to use.

Interactivity can be more difficult in traditional tiered lecture theatres but it is still possible to ask people to talk to their immediate neighbours (side, behind) for short periods of time. The important thing to remember is that how you react to your environment – in terms of minimizing its limitations – can make a difference to how useful your learners see the session. This emphasizes the importance of arriving early in order to see if you need to make adjustments in order to maximize your impact.

Light is of particular importance, especially when using PowerPoint. Try the lights on various settings until you find the one that balances your visibility with most readable screen views.

Set

An essential prerequisite of set is, of course, preparation and it is probably a useful rule of thumb that you need to spend at least the same time on preparation as you do on presentation. This is more so, the more advanced the technology you employ. However, it does have the advantage that having once given a lecture, you have a sound basis for a future presentation.

Once all environmental concerns have been met, you should be ready to begin your lecture.

The Advanced Trauma Life Support (ATLS), in their most recent version of the instructor course, considered the following acronym to be helpful:[4]

A	Attention	Welcoming students; introducing yourself; claiming credibility
I	Interest	Establishing motivation; laying claims to value of session and contribution towards the course as a whole
D	Direction	Best provided by title and learning outcome slides
S	Student involvement	Explaining how students will be involved: asking and answering questions, activities, etc.

At other times, others have suggested attention to:[5]
- mood;
- motivation;
- objectives;
- roles.

Or, supported by an acronym:[6]
- roles;
- objectives;
- motivation;
- atmosphere;

all of which cover similar territory, in slightly different words. Whichever words are used to describe this part of the session, it is an essential component of a successful lecture, providing the audience with the opportunity to 'tune in' to what is going to follow. A lecture that does not cover this territory is at risk of not giving students the best opportunity to learn from the dialogue that follows.

Let us explore the ATLS acronym in more detail.

Gaining attention. Your first words should be to welcome your audience and to say a little about who you are, even if you have been introduced. It is not immodest to say who you are or to claim some expertise in the subject matter under consideration. However, resist making grandiose claims (e.g. future Nobel prize winner).

Establishing interest. It is valuable to make a general statement of the aim(s) of the session and to indicate the intended learning outcomes. During this part of the set it is useful to indicate the extent to which the material is relevant to the needs of the audience and to perhaps suggest its importance.

Direction. Learning outcomes can here be more helpful than objectives, often thought of as vague and ill-defined. The characteristics of learning outcomes have been summarized as follows:[7]

> [They] should be expressed through the use of active verbs which spell out what students will be able to do. In order to achieve clarity, expressions such as 'to know', 'to understand', 'to appreciate', 'to be acquainted with', should be avoided, since they are too vague to convey the exact nature of the outcome being sought. More active and explicit verbs such as 'state', 'show', 'explain', 'define', 'describe', 'predict', 'recognise' and 'criticise' should be used wherever possible.

While learning outcomes often lay the basis for assessment, the lecture does not normally enable that. However, the audience can make personal judgements as to the extent to which they feel they have met the outcomes at the end of the lecture. If they have not, they should know where they need to rectify their deficit.

Student involvement. It can be helpful to let your audience know what is expected of them: you may want to indicate that you will ask them some questions (see below); to involve them in small group or pair-based discussions; you may want to tell them that they can ask questions, or save these for the end of your session.

An aside: more on questions
This was explored in some detail in Chapter 2 but it is worth reiterating aspects of that in the context of the lecture. Remember that questions of the learners can be key elements of a successful lecture, in order to:[4]
• gain and maintain attention;
• assess levels of understanding;
• increase levels of understanding;
• increase buy-in;
• increase mutual learning.
However, there are some strategies to avoid:
• lengthy questions;
• questions within questions;
• ambiguous questions;
• too many questions;
• fixating;
• flirting.
The first four of these are relatively obvious, but fixating and flirting need further exploration.

Fixating. This is where the lecturer, having found a willing respondent to earlier questions, looks to that person for future answers, thereby depriving other members of the audience from the opportunity to participate.

Flirting... is the reverse, where a member of the audience seeks approval from the lecturer by asking questions and gaining his/her interest. You may be sceptical about this, mainly because it can be flattering to have someone express admiration and interest in your ideas but it is based on something that Brookfield[8] described as: 'an emotional battleground with members vying for recognition and affirmation from each other and from the [lecturer].'

There are a variety of ways, with advantages and disadvantages, in which lecturers can ask questions of their audience.

ACTIVITY 3.3

Complete the table below:

Asking questions of …	Advantages	Disadvantages
A row		
Named individual		
Whole audience		
Random individuals		
Pose, pause, pounce*		

See end of chapter for response.

Dialogue

It is almost a statement of the obvious that the dialogue is the opportunity to 'tell them'† – in other words, provide the substance of your content. However, there are a number of important provisos as to how you might go about doing this.

First, your presentation must be in the right order: you are not going to be presenting a series of random facts or points of view, but you must tell the story and unravel the plot. This is an important distinction and one that the novelist, critic and academic, E.M. Forster drew attention to:[9]

> We have defined a story as a narrative of events arranged in their time-sequence. A plot is also a narrative of events, the emphasis falling on causality. 'The king died and then the queen died,' is a story. 'The king died, and then the queen died of grief' is a plot. The time sequence is preserved, but the sense of causality overshadows it … If it is in a story we say 'and then?' If it is in a plot we ask 'why'?

In a great deal of CME, time sequencing is an important component: indeed, it is essential in all of the life support group programmes working within, for example, ABCDE type protocols.

It is this element of lecturing that justifies the description 'dialogue': however, the dialogue in this case is (on the whole, but see interactive lectures

---

*This approach involves: (1) asking question; (2) pausing (5 seconds or so) and (3) asking a named individual for a response.

† 'Tell them what you are going to tell them, tell them, tell them what you have told them' – numerous sources.

below) one way in terms of public discourse, but there is, it is hoped, consideration of story and plot taking place in the heads of the audience. You may well have told your audience that you will be engaging with them through questions and answers but it is worth considering more deliberate attempts to engage them through the use of interactive lectures.

Interactive lectures

Interactive lectures can range from a lecture with lots of questions, usually from the lecturer to the audience, or more structured interaction among small groups in the audience. The obvious place to introduce interactivity is 10–15 minutes into a lecture when attention starts to wane. However, if it is your first time giving a lecture, the advice is to keep it simple as these techniques can be challenging initially.

Ways of introducing interactivity
Electronic voting systems/Ask the audience. Some institutions issue students with alpha numeric pads so that they can be monitored for attendance as well as formative learning. These can be a great way to introduce interactivity as most systems come with their own software which can produce instant graphics, how many answered, what button they pressed and basic statistics comparing with previous answers – personally and in the group. For example, a question can be asked and if the majority do not answer the question correctly, the lecturer can clarify misunderstandings. This system has been introduced in one university where the failure rate at the end of the course has significantly reduced. As well as formatively testing knowledge, they are good for seeking opinions from the group and introducing concepts. Even without high technology, a show of hands can be a useful way of introducing interactivity.

Buzz groups. This is where you ask the audience to discuss a question in groups (usually pairs in a tiered lecture theatre, or fours if they can turn around and speak to those behind them). The opportunity then arises for you to go around and observe groups, facilitate ones that are appear stuck but generally to enjoy the happy sound of an interactive lecture (Fig. 3.2). This emphasizes the social needs of learners and helps them see other people's points of view. Each group feeds back to the larger group.

Brainstorming. This form of interactivity is good for the first time you meet and helps break the ice. It also helps to generate ideas and themes at the beginning of a course. Contextual examples include asking a question of the audience, who then give you a range of answers, which can be blocked together in themes in order to fit the structure of the rest of your lecture. An example of this might be as follows.

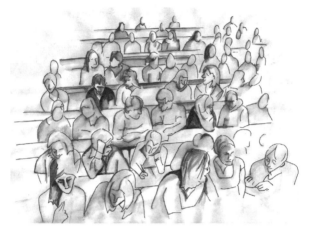

Figure 3.2 An interactive lecture

You ask the question: 'What concerns would you have when a child was brought into emergency department following a road traffic accident?' and you receive the following answers:

1 Can the child talk to me?
2 Are there obvious signs of bleeding?
3 Does she have a surgical collar on?
4 Is there a senior in the department?
5 When I look at her, can I see her chest moving?
6 Are her parents here?

Your flip chart may look like this (see Chapter 2):

Airway
Breathing
Circulation
Other

and, as you get responses, you fill in the gaps in the order you receive them, thus the following:

Airway	Circulation
Can the child talk to me	Are there obvious signs of bleeding?
Does she have a surgical collar on?	
Breathing	Other
When I look at her, can I see her chest moving?	Is there a senior in the department? Are her parents here?

You may find the need to paraphrase what someone says and all answers and solutions should be considered. The emphasis is on not discounting anything, perhaps even accommodating apparently unconventional or irrelevant ideas, for example:

What kind of car was it that hit her?

This might have significance for thinking about mechanism of injury.

Interactive handouts. Leaving blanks on your handouts that the audience have to fill in at the appropriate time. For example, the derivation of an equation, thinking of a list of causes or working out a dose of medication. The answer can be revealed during the lecture or given at your next meeting.

Any of these, but particularly apparently 'tutorless activities' might seem to be a somewhat risky strategy and may raise questions such as:

- Will I lose control?
- Will I achieve the intended learning outcomes?
- Will the audience do what I ask them to do?
- Will they be able to do it in the time available?

It is worth taking each of these in turn.

Will I lose control? I have argued elsewhere in this book (Chapters 1 and 4) that control is rarely something you need to worry about. However, there are some technical issues, and these are about how you gain attention once you have lively discussion going on in the lecture theatre. There are a number of options.

ACTIVITY 3.4

Can you think of any?. *See end of chapter for response.*

Will I achieve the intended learning outcomes? There are two stages in this: first, making clear what the learning outcomes are by drawing attention to them in your set; second, by emphasizing important issues in your summary (see Closure below).

Will the audience do what I ask them to do? If they understand the task, they will. There may be some temporary resistance but experience shows that they will concur with requests made of them. It is important in order to avoid 'dependency' and this can be done by having the instructions written on a flip chart or PowerPoint slide. Groups often will delay a start by asking 'What should we be doing?' or similar requests, and these are trying to avoid 'work' (in Bion's terms; see Chapter 1).

Will they be able to do the work in the time available? This is a risk associated with interactive activities and time management is important, particularly when there are a number of sessions with other speakers. It is your responsibility to know when to interrupt, gather some feedback from the groups who have been exploring the issues you have set them and giving opportun-ities for asking questions before you summarize.

Tutorless groups raise the greatest level of anxiety in setting up interactive sessions but they can be powerful sources of learning. One of the most important considerations is that the groups are left to work on their own. If you join groups, or hover over them, you will change the dynamic and they will look to you for answers rather than seeking the answers for themselves.

An aside on jokes

Unless you are a talented performer, do not tell them: you may forget the punchline or get it wrong and have to start again. However, it is perfectly acceptable to be witty if it is in your normal conversational repertoire. Humorous slides (Larson cartoons are a favourite) can contribute as long as they are pertinent and funny. Try them out on people who will tell you the truth.

Closure

Closure is an important element in a lecture in that it allows you to bring things together through two main processes.

Questions

When you have finished your dialogue, it is important to ask an audience if they have any questions or comments. If you are using a PowerPoint projector, it is worth putting in a question slide to remind you to do this (Fig. 3.3).

Summary

As explored in Chapter 2, you will then summarize, revisiting your learning outcomes and leaving your audience with a clear take home message. This might include important emphasis or content that arose from questions.

Up to this point in this chapter, the focus has been on the content and the organization – to a large extent the intended 'message'. In the final section, we need to consider aspects of 'the medium'.[10]

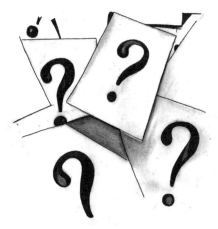

Figure 3.3 Any questions?

Some teaching courses offer the opportunity to be videoed during a short 10-minute teaching session and to be critiqued by a performance coach. This is invaluable in seeing your own shortcomings (one of mine was hand-wringing – I was advised to carry something, such as a pointer, to help me stop doing it). It is also very useful to have another person, perhaps someone who is not medical and therefore less threatening, to give you feedback on personal aspects that may not annoy you but do annoy everyone else. Another way of doing this is to be peer assessed during your teaching.

Many of the potential pitfalls have their origins in verbal and non-verbal ways of communicating, as opposed to content, and these issues are discussed below.

Verbal style
There are a number of considerations that you need to focus on.

Voice
You cannot do very much about aspects of your vocal presentation (e.g. pitch is determined by gender and your genes and the different physiology that arise from these). Accent also may, at least to some extent, be determined by an individual's background 'community of practice' (see Chapter 1). However, it is true that people who have been exposed to varieties of accent tend to drift towards a type of undifferentiated standard English accent. Slight regional varieties may still expose themselves but do not interfere with effective communication.

Rate

The rate of delivery is inversely proportionate to the levels of understanding that the audience can reasonably be expected to achieve: the faster the delivery, the less understanding, either of individual words and phrases or the sense of the subject under discussion. An ideal rate is something slightly slower than normal conversation. This gives time for the audience to take in the message and to begin to integrate what they are hearing with what they already know. If an audience experiences a fast delivery, they will quickly tune out and hope that the lecture ends soon: it will, leaving a gap in the programme.

Modulation

Your lecture should possess the patterns of intonation that normal speech possesses, neither more nor less. Less suggests an alien invader, more implies a Joyce Grenfell type of primary school teacher, which inevitably sounds patronizing.

Emphasis

Some parts of your lecture may require emphasis and this can be achieved through a number of strategies:
- Slowing down
- Repetition
- 'What I am going to say next is particularly important …'

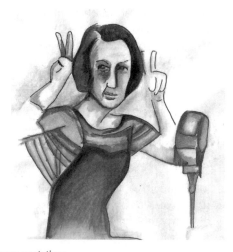

Figure 3.4 Finger quotations

One strategy to avoid, however, is the finger quotation mark (Fig. 3.4) which has an amazing capacity to annoy an audience.

Redundancy

Some redundancy (e.g. repetition for emphasis or as part of a micro summary) can contribute towards audience understanding. However, spoken languages have two types of 'hesitation phenomena': silent pauses and filled pauses. Both are easy to spot by an audience, the former by hesitancy and the latter by such fillers as 'er', 'um', 'OK', 'Do you get me?' Both can become very distracting: a talented and otherwise articulate lecturer was found to have used 148 'OKs' in a 45-minute lecture. That the number was counted is an indication of the extent to which they can be distracting.

Enthusiasm

It almost goes without saying that you have to be interested in what you are saying and to demonstrate this through the animation of your delivery. If you are bored, your audience will certainly be the same, shortly after you manifest a desire to be somewhere else. Even if you have delivered the same lecture many times, remind yourself why you thought it was interesting the first time you heard or presented it. If you cannot replicate this, it might be better for your reputation that you suggest an alternative. This is a great way of spreading the load. As you take on more and more responsibilities, pressures build up and I have personally handed over lectures to other colleagues to develop. At first this was very hard – like letting your baby go – but then a relief as you see the topic grow with new input.

Non-verbal style

Once more, there are a number of issues.

Body language

You may have heard of the three elements of communication – and the '7%–38%–55% Mehrabian rule'. In his studies, Mehrabian came to the conclusion that there are basically three elements in any face-to-face communication: words, tone of voice and body language. He assigned varying percentages of association with these elements (7% to words, 38% to tone of voice and 55% to body language) as to whether you liked the person speaking. However, some people claim that in any communication situation, the meaning of a message was conveyed mainly by non-verbal cues, not by the meaning of words. This generalization, from an initially very specific condition in his experiment, is the basic mistake around the misinterpretation of the Mehrabian rule.

Nevertheless, it is safe to argue that as listeners, we are affected by a range of behaviours that can interfere with the overt message. We have already discussed tone of voice and as well as the capacity of that to undermine understanding, body language also has significant impact. Behaviour such as elaborate gesturing, striding up and down, jingling coins and car keys in pockets or clicking pens can be very distracting.

Proximity

Equally, positioning is important, particularly if there is a rostrum, lectern or table. Being behind one of these could suggest you are trying to hide from your audience. Similarly, aggressive striding up and down in front of (or into) the audience can be off-putting. Avoid getting too close to members of the audience in the front row as you communicate with individuals towards the back. You need to establish where you feel comfortable (but not in sight lines), and where you feel you can maintain close contact with your audience.

Eye contact

Last but not least is eye contact: the responsibility for maintaining this is yours. In the first instance you will have lots of attention from your audience and all you need to do is to continually sweep the room, even if the auditorium is in darkness: your posture in that circumstance will suggest that it is something you are striving for.

The audience's eyes can tell you a great deal: from complete interest to deep sleep. Hopefully, if you use the techniques described above, they will never reach this state.

3.4 Conclusions

Remember the ABCDE of lecturing. Do not:[11]
• annoy;
• bore;
• confuse;
• distract;
• exhaust.

References

1 Anon. *Change Theories: Pedagogy of the Oppressed by Paulo Freire – An Analysis.* 2003. http://www.comminit.com/changetheories/ctheories/changetheories-41. html [accessed on 19 August 2006]

2 Stuart J, Rutherford R. Medical student concentration during lectures. *Lancet* 1978;2:514–516.

3 Benedict M, Hoag J. Seating location in large lectures: Are seating preferences or location related to course performance? *Journal of Economics Education* 2004;35:215–231.

4 American College of Surgeons Committee on Trauma. *ATLS Student Course Manual* (7th edn.) 2004. American College of Surgeons, Chicago.

5 Mackway-Jones K, Walker M. *Pocket Guide to Teaching for Medical Instructors.* 1999. BMJ Books, London.

6 ALSG slide set, 2004.

7 Sackville A. Writing learning outcomes: A guide. http://www.edgehill.ac.uk/tld/staff/b1/outcomes.htm [Accessed on 5 July 2006]

8 Brookfield S. Through the lens of learning: How the visceral experience of learning reframes teaching. In Boud D, Cohen R, Walker D. (eds.) *Using Experience for Learning.* 1993. SRHE/Open University Press, Buckingham.

9 Forster EM. *Aspects of the Novel.* (1927/2005). Penguin, Harmondsworth.

10 McLuhan M. *Understanding Media: The Extensions of Man.* 1964/2001. Routledge, London. [McLuhan believed that the content was much less important than its method of delivery; see Activity 3.1.]

11 Acland R. A In Dent J, Harden R. (eds.) Lectures (Chapter 6). *Practical Guide for Medical Teachers.* 2001. Churchill Livingstone, London: p.67.

Responses to activities

Activity 3.1

Everyone reading this book will have heard, during the course of their studies, countless lectures. It is almost inevitable that few, if any, have stuck in readers' minds. However, you may be able to recall an experience of the lecturer.

Therefore, you may find that you wrote things such as:

• a charismatic lecturer;
• use of humour;
• committed and enthusiastic lecturer;
• entertaining.

It is rare when this question is asked that people talk about content; they are far more likely to talk about the qualities of the lecturer and the extent to which they have been entertained rather than informed. Indeed, it is a rare event when a lecturer tells an audience something that is new to them. Most audiences are familiar with the territory, if not in detail at least in context. Even when audiences are hearing something completely new (e.g. Darwin's theories of evolution) there has usually been some kind of debate in the public domain in advance of the lecture itself.

Activity 3.2

A/V aid	Pros	Cons
Black/whiteboard	Interactive; dynamic	Handwriting; spelling; time
Overhead projector	Can edit your presentation on the fly; can be well designed – it is hard to produce a bad slide if you use default settings (e.g. in PowerPoint)	Old technology; bulbs; poor presentation (e.g. busy slides, handwritten notes)
Flip chart	Interactive; dynamic; permanent	Handwriting; spelling; time
35-mm slide projector	High quality; good for clinical slides	Old technology; bulbs
Video/DVD player	Can animate; good for clinical demonstrations	Passive; DVDs more difficult to cue
Computer + data projector	High quality design; access to multimedia (e.g. use of reusable learning objects; interactive (to a degree))	Equipment failure
Interactive whiteboard	Wide range of applications (capable of anything a PC can do, including link to printer)	Initial set-up costs + ongoing costs (projector bulbs very expensive); some training required

Activity 3.3

Asking questions of ...	Advantages	Disadvantages
A row	Can ensure all get asked	Early responders can go 'off duty', late responders experience anxiety as the options disappear
Named individual	Keeps audience alert	Can cause high anxiety (thereby diminishing ability to respond)
Whole audience	Less pressure	No one may answer
Random individuals	It may serve to keep the audience awake	Some people may not be asked and may feel relieved or deprived
Pose, pause, pounce	Gives everyone an opportunity to frame a response	Similar to asking a named individual

Activity 3.4

You might have thought of any of these:

- clapping your hands;
- ringing a bell;
- shouting;
- standing up;
- walking round groups letting them know they have 2 minutes;
- beginning to speak.

I feel strongly that the first four of these (especially shouting) are inappropriate for adult – and for that matter – child audiences. Standing up can work but depends on you being seen to alter your position. Giving advanced warning of closure can work in certain settings but not with large groups, particularly those in tiered lecture theatres. My personal preference is beginning to speak – talking inconsequentially about your journey that day, for example. The groups nearest to you think you are saying something important and go quiet; their silence is 'heard' by neighbouring groups and this spreads rapidly backwards, at which point you have regained attention.

Chapter 4 **Workshops and discussion groups**

The purpose of this chapter is to explore the contribution of workshops and discussion groups (small groups) of various kinds to continuing medical education (CME).

4.1 Learning outcomes

The learning outcomes for this chapter are to:
• identify opportunities and challenges of workshops and discussion groups;
• describe the varied characteristics of different types of workshops and discussion groups;
• describe how to manage the variety of workshops and discussion groups;
• recognize strategies;
• facilitate the tutorless group.

Chapter 1 explored some of the theory underlying behaviour in groups. The purpose of this chapter is to examine how that can be realized in practice and how an instructor can ease the process for the learners.

Why small groups?
Small groups have a taken for grantedness about them that it is worth exploring.

ACTIVITY 4.1

What justifications would you use for using small group teaching? *See end of chapter for response.*

How to Teach Continuing Medical Education. By Mike Davis and Kirsty Forrest. Published 2008 by Blackwell Publishing. ISBN: 978-1-4051-5398-0

ACTIVITY 4.2

What are your fears about running small group discussions? *See end of chapter for response.*

Small group work is not appropriate for all of your learners' needs but by choosing the right issues and laying appropriate foundations, learners can get a great deal from them.

There are a number of issues that need to be considered before choosing to run a group discussion:

1 How many learners will I be working with?
2 What are the interpersonal issues I will have to deal with?
3 What kind of space is available?
  • Is the furniture fixed or portable?
  • What kind of layout shall I use?
  • Is there any audiovisual equipment?

Group size

Discussion groups are rarely successful with more than 12 participants and, depending on the nature of the task, 4–6 might be more appropriate. If numbers exceed 12, it will be necessary to initiate what would almost certainly happen anyway – the establishment of sub-groups who then function in a more tutorless way. This will be explored in more detail later in this chapter.

Interpersonal issues

The role of the instructor is more of a facilitator during these sessions. This means that you should listen much more than you talk. After your initial statement, you should, through subtle use of body language and a particular approach to asking questions (see below), allow the conversation to develop among the candidates, having them speaking to one another rather than directing everything to you. This saves you from occupying a 'judicial' role, which is something that can be observed in adult education settings where sessions become, 'Emotional battlegrounds with members vying for recognition and affirmation from each other and from the discussion leader.'[1]

This is the socioemotional component of the learning environment and, unless it is well handled, can interfere with effective learning for many group members. More significant, however, is the nature of the interactions that are expected among the group. The question we should consider is, 'What is the nature of the intellectual activity that candidates are engaging in?' In lectures, this is relatively straightforward: candidates listen, consider, compare with existing knowledge and either accept or reject the conclusions – usually the former. In discussion, however, it is not simply a matter of rehearsing what has been previously read. As Candy puts it:[2]

> If cognitive process are indeed processes of reconstruction rather than replicating or depicting an a priori existing reality, then the focus of any explanatory effort must shift from what there is or may be to how we arrive at the conceptual constructs we actually have.

Space
Clearly, you need sufficient space to seat everyone comfortably. If you are given a very large space, it is preferable to use a corner and, if possible, use lighting to help close down the surplus areas. People do not like to find themselves in the centre of large well-lit spaces as it makes them feel overlooked.

It is not impossible that you find yourself in a lecture theatre with fixed, possibly tiered seating. In these circumstances it is still possible to put together a group of about 6–8 in a degree of comfort. Let participants work it out for themselves: some individuals resist being told where and how to sit.

In general, the layout for a discussion group is more 'democratic' than for a lecture. Apart from the size of the group it is more likely to encourage closer proximity and mutual eye contact. Conventional arrangements are as follows.

It would be useful in the first instance to distinguish among the different types of group and the following table may help to raise some of the issues:

	Closed discussion	Workshop	Open discussion
Questions and answers	Through the instructor	Of one another	Of one another
Nature of dialogue	Mainly closed questions to identified individuals	Open questions (mainly), after initial direction	Open questions, after initial direction
Arrangement	Horseshoe	Depends on content of workshop (see equipment)	Circle
Equipment	A/V	A/V; clinical equipment; clinical information	None

(Continued)

	Closed discussion	Workshop	Open discussion
Role of instructor	Direction of discussion; summary	Introduction; redirection; error correction; summary	Introduction (micro summaries + redirection); summary
Subject matter	Known answer to problem (e.g. triage discussion)	Mainly known – but applying procedures and protocols to novel case information (e.g. reading rhythm strips)	Not necessarily any right answers (e.g. discussion of ethical issues informed by good practice)

For ease of reference, the remainder of this chapter focuses on each type of discussion in turn.

4.2 Closed discussion groups

Closed discussion groups have a great deal in common with interactive lectures in that they are moving towards a predetermined end where the instructor knows the correct answers. More often than not, these groups involve a smaller number of learners than a lecture: 4–6 being not uncommon. They are often supported by flip charts and/or overhead projectors or computer projection and the usual arrangement is a horseshoe with the facilitator sitting next to the A/V aid(s) in the open jaws (Fig. 4.1).

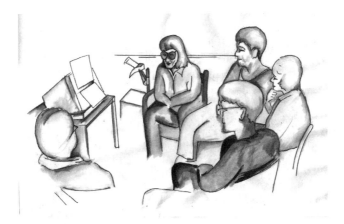

Figure 4.1 Discussion groups

In the horseshoe, candidates can still have eye contact with one another and attention can be drawn to the screen whenever the instructor wants to regain control over the direction of the session.

As part of your preparation of your environment, ensure that your equipment works and that you are familiar with managing transitions from slide to slide. Other environmental concerns are explored in Chapter 2.

The particular role of the facilitator in a closed discussion is to ask appropriate questions and, as was explored in Chapter 2, there is a helpful hierarchy to work with. In the following section, we work through an exemplar closed discussion based on the following triage scenario.

You are summoned to a triage area at a camping site where five holidaymakers are injured in a gas explosion in a caravan. After you quickly survey the situation, the patients' conditions are as follows:

Patient A: A young woman is screaming, 'Please help me, my chest hurts.'

Patient B: An 8-year-old boy is cyanotic, tachypneic and breathing very noisily.

Patient C: An elderly man is lying in a pool of blood with his left trouser leg soaked in blood. He is moaning.

Patient D: A middle-aged woman is lying face down on a stretcher and not moving.

Patient E: A young man is swearing and shouting that someone should help him or he will call his lawyer.

Set

Assuming you have paid attention to your environment and you have introduced yourself and the group, you now need to begin to explore the topic. You might say something like:

Instructor: I know you have read this before, but just take a minute to refresh your memory about this scenario.

Make sure you give the minute: it might be a good idea to time yourself.

ACTIVITY 4.3

Think about your first question.

The question cues you should be thinking of here belong in the *knowledge* category so a key verb might be: list, define, tell, describe, identify, show, label, collect, examine, tabulate, quote, name, who, when, where.

What would be a good opening question? *See end of chapter for response.*

This question will enable the candidates to focus on the essential heuristic: A, B, C, D and E.

You may have already prepared a flip chart page with a matrix, as follows:

	Airway	Breathing	Circulation	Disability	Exposure
Patient A					
Patient B					
Patient C					
Patient D					
Patient E					

and the group can now work together to identify issues for each patient in turn and thereby enable them to make a decision based on clinical need:

OK, who can *identify* what is wrong with patient A? Does she have an airway problem?

You may want to ask a few more knowledge-based questions to ensure that the group have grasped the essential nature of the task. It is not useful, at this stage, to ask questions like, 'Does everyone understand?' as it is extremely unlikely that anyone will own up to not understanding, even if they do not.

Essentially, this first phase is one of information processing: in other words, data (i.e. clinical signs) is being converted into meaningful information.

The next level of questioning is designed to engage at the level of *comprehension* and some question cues include: summarize, describe, interpret, contrast, predict, associate, distinguish, estimate, differentiate, discuss, extend. A helpful question might be:

Can anyone *describe* patient A's state in relation to the ABCs?

Or, somewhat further down the line:

How would you *distinguish* patient A's needs from those of patient D?

Much of this discussion is going to take place at these levels, although if there was a moral or ethical dimension to a decision it might achieve the level of evaluation, when a possible question would be:

Can you *explain* why you think that more attention needs paying to an 8-year-old boy than an elderly man?

There could be a point at which this conversation takes on some of the appearance of an open discussion if it is sensitively handled. This would require the instructor to sit back (literally and figuratively) and enable the exchange to take place among candidates for as long as it was productive. How you might do this is dealt with later in this chapter.

As with all teaching sessions, a closed discussion needs to come to a conclusion and given that there is a 'right' answer to the question that is posed, the need for this should emerge when the group has explored all of the issues it needs to address. At this point the instructor should offer the group the opportunity to make any additional comments or ask any questions that are specific to the approach (in this case, using a matrix to explore triage). Following that opportunity, the instructor should summarize all aspects of the discussion, including both the process (the matrix as a tool for assisting the decision-making process; the application of ABCDE principles) and the decision itself. Candidates can then be told what they will be doing next.

4.3 Workshops

A workshop has similarities with both the closed discussion described above and also with the lecture, explored in detail in Chapter 3, and these similarities will become apparent in this section.

The purpose of the workshop is to give detailed consideration to knowledge and skills in an environment where it is safe and appropriate to acknowledge doubt and uncertainty, and to resolve these before being faced with the reality of work-based practice.

The workshop can go beyond clinical skills teaching (see Chapter 5) and may include aspects of psychomotor skill as part of an exploration of wider issues dominated by knowledge, understanding and application. In terms of the Miller[3] hierarchy, the workshop provides 'knows how' opportunities to candidates, with the potential for some simulated 'shows how' using manikins or role players. The discussion may be supported by the use of audiovisual aids (often overhead projector and transparencies) and some equipment – for learners to gain familiarity, rather than practising use. A workshop might look something like Fig. 4.2.

Examples of the structure of workshops include:
• directed cases;
• role play (in certain contexts; see Chapter 6).
  In the context of subjects such as:
• blood gas analysis;
• interpreting electrocardiogram (ECG) output;
• pain management.

Temporal sequences can be managed by introducing additional information as and when progress is being made, by adding new slides or revealing new information. For example, when using case-based scenarios additional

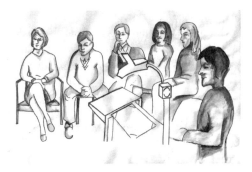

Figure 4.2 A workshop

information can be introduced when a particular stage has been reached or to help out when a problem is encountered.

An aside on 'strippers' and 'flashers'
The use of overhead transparencies, particularly, have the capacity to annoy half an audience by the choice you make between being a stripper or a flasher.

A flasher reveals the whole content of a slide at the same time, whereas a stripper reveals a little bit at a time. Apart from the audience reaction, they have their advantages and disadvantages:

	Advantages	Disadvantages
Stripper	Timely introduction of new information Leads to predetermined conclusions	Can accidentally reveal information Does not allow for novel interpretations or solutions Slide handling can be clumsy
Flasher	Audience can see everything from the beginning No need to handle slides	May give away crucial information (e.g. a diagnosis)

Another alternative to stripping when it is necessary to have sequential additions of new information is to produce multiple slides with additional information in each.

The workshop is designed to increase the confidence of learners in applying theoretical principles (cognition) and moving towards clinical competence (behaviour) in simulated or work-based settings.

The role of the instructor is particularly important and indeed the role may be conceived of differently when working in this more interactive environment. In Chapter 1, there was frequent reference to the word 'facilitator' and this is often the role taken in workshops and discussions. The word has its origins in the notion of making things easy (i.e. facile), but more recent connotations are more likely to refer to the process of enabling or developing the capacity for empowerment. This has a significant impact on the way in which the instructor behaves, particularly at the beginning of a session, and on the type of questions that might be asked.

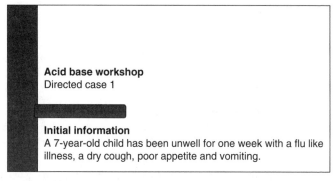

Acid base workshop
Directed case 1

Initial information
A 7-year-old child has been unwell for one week with a flu like illness, a dry cough, poor appetite and vomiting.

Figure 4.3 Acid base workshop: directed case. Reproduced with kind permission of Advanced Life Support Group.

An example – Acid base workshop: directed case

Clearly, the opening remarks (set) will follow the conventions explored in Chapter 2 but from then on, the role is to pose an opening statement that will allow the learners to begin to share their existing knowledge in order to have a clearer understanding of the issues and to move towards reaching quite complex clinical decisions. The opening statement needs to provide relevant clinical information and a question at the level of *analysis* in Bloom's taxonomy, based on the desire to establish:
• identification of components;
• patterns and associations.

'Can you *explore* what your thinking might be on being presented with this initial information?' might be a useful starting point.

The discussion will, at this point, be quite tentative as there is not much in the history or presentation to go on. However, when new information arrives, the discussion can be redirected (Fig. 4.4).

At this point, the role of the facilitator changes quite significantly from being somewhat centre stage, to observing quietly. Using a description often

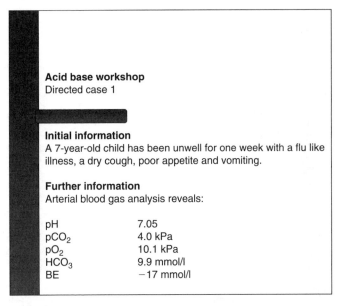

Acid base workshop
Directed case 1

Initial information
A 7-year-old child has been unwell for one week with a flu like illness, a dry cough, poor appetite and vomiting.

Further information
Arterial blood gas analysis reveals:

pH	7.05
pCO_2	4.0 kPa
pO_2	10.1 kPa
HCO_3	9.9 mmol/l
BE	−17 mmol/l

Figure 4.4 More information is given

used in discussions of facilitating online learning, the change in role is from 'the sage on the stage' (i.e. the fount of all knowledge) to 'the guide on the side' (i.e. providing additional information and prompts, as and when the need arises). In presenting the further information, a question that might be asked could be: 'What would you *infer* from this arterial blood gas analysis?' In practical terms, what the facilitator can now do is to stand somewhat to one side and to disengage from actively contributing to the discussion. While actively listening to the discussion, the facilitator should avoid eye contact with anyone in the group thereby encouraging them to address their remarks to one another. This issue of eye contact will be explored more fully later in the chapter.

At the point at which learners need the final set of information (Fig. 4.5), the facilitator can make it available (by stripping or putting up a new, now complete, slide) and asking a question, at the level of *synthesis*: '*What if* you take this following information into account?' and then retiring once more to an inobtrusive but observant position while the new information is *integrated*. The discussion, at this point, might be confirming of initial impressions or challenging those. The group reaching a decision, or consensus, would be the end of the dialogue phase of the workshop at which point the

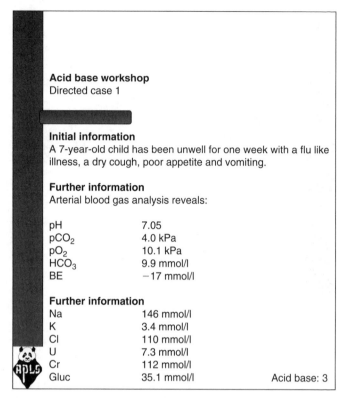

Acid base workshop
Directed case 1

Initial information
A 7-year-old child has been unwell for one week with a flu like illness, a dry cough, poor appetite and vomiting.

Further information
Arterial blood gas analysis reveals:

pH	7.05
pCO_2	4.0 kPa
pO_2	10.1 kPa
HCO_3	9.9 mmol/l
BE	−17 mmol/l

Further information
Na	146 mmol/l
K	3.4 mmol/l
Cl	110 mmol/l
U	7.3 mmol/l
Cr	112 mmol/l
Gluc	35.1 mmol/l

Acid base: 3

Figure 4.5 And more information is given

facilitator returns to centre stage and initiates closure, by asking for questions or comments and offering a summary.

4.4 Open discussion

The open discussion invariably takes place with all participants, including the facilitator, sitting in a circle – as far as possible the chairs should be the same so that no one looks like a group leader, as in Fig. 4.6.

The open discussion is often the modality that causes the greatest anxiety, largely because of the facilitator's fear of losing control. However, this is unfounded as there are easy strategies for controlling even the most difficult situation in the unlikely event that one would arise. However, as was explored in Chapter 1, groups have a capacity to avoid sophisticated behaviour (i.e. work) and engage instead in varieties of task avoidance unless they are facilitated effectively.

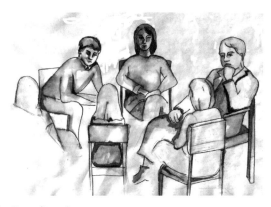

Figure 4.6 Open discussion group

Before effective facilitation is explored, just a reminder of how groups can avoid their task:

Strategy	Associated behaviours
Dependency	Asking for confirmation about the nature of the task Asking for clarification Checking for affirmation (from facilitator and other group members) Seeking approval
Flight	Talking off task Telling jokes Describing work title/practices

Fight	Complaining about:
	  the task
	  aspects of the environment
	  the programme
	  the facilitator

Pairing	Giving way to dominant members Off-task fascination Argumentative behaviour/personal attacks on other group members

The role of the facilitator is to tolerate aspects of this: seeing it as a natural function of how groups work, rather than a threat to authority. However, there are a number of conditions that an effective facilitator can exploit in order to ensure that the group engages in 'work', as this table illustrates:

Behaviour	Response
Asking for confirmation about the nature of the task	Making a clear and unambiguous statement in your opening comment but having it written up on a screen or flip chart can help
Asking for clarification	Saying something like 'As you see it'
Checking for affirmation (from facilitator and other group members)	Initiating the discussion, saying something like 'Tell us what you think'
Seeking approval	Saying something like 'What do others think?'
Talking off task	Inviting a direct response from the talker
Telling jokes	Acknowledging, laughing (if funny), and moving on: 'So ...' to other side of circle
Describing work title/practices	Saying 'Tell us how [...] fits with your experience'
Complaining about: the task	Ignoring*
aspects of the environment	Asking the group 'Are you warm/cool enough?' and making environmental adjustments if appropriate
the programme	Ignoring
the facilitator	Ignoring
Giving way to dominant members	Asking for comments
Off-task fascination	Summarizing and redirecting
Argumentative behaviour/personal attacks on other group members	Closing down the argumentative person

Much of the work of managing an open discussion is in what you do, rather than what you say.

Some experts in communication argue that body language communicates more than words. Certainly, some unconscious behaviours can communicate

---

* This might feel like a high-risk strategy, but on the whole, people will want to ignore these comments and challenging them will almost certainly involve a dialogue which will guarantee that the task will not be completed. It is highly likely that the rest of the group will follow your example.

very effectively and particular attention needs to be paid to these to avoid negative impact on the group. Some helpful strategies include:

- Making frequent sweeps of the group at eye level but not giving eye contact to a person who is speaking. This might sound hostile or aggressive but it makes people speak to the group rather than to you.
- Sitting back after your initial statement and subsequent questions.

Not validating (nodding, saying 'excellent') contributions – this will encourage the group to believe they have found the 'right' answer and the discussion will have come to an end without all candidates having had time to contribute and to think it through. Again this may feel uncomfortable but it does encourage the group to continue to explore the issues.

ACTIVITY 4.4

Have another look at Fig. 4.6. Who is leading this group? *See end of chapter for response.*

4.5 Conclusions

Small groups lay bare some of the complex sociopsychological issues of teaching and learning, mainly arising from instructors' concerns about power and authority. However, much of the research suggests that among fairly well-motivated communities, group cohesion and a sense of responsibility almost guarantee the status quo (i.e. the instructor is the site of power in the group and all group members subscribe to that because of their psychological need for safety).

References

1 Brookfield S. Through the lens of learning: How the visceral experience of learning reframes teaching. In Boud D, Cohen R, Walker D. (eds.) *Using Experience for Learning.* 1993. SHRE/Open University, Buckingham: p. 24.

2 Candy P. *Self-direction for Lifelong Learning.* 1991. Jossey-Bass, San Francisco, CA: p. 273.

3 Miller G. The assessment of clinical skills/competence/performance. *Academic Medicine* 1990;**65**:563–567.

Responses to activities

Activity 4.1

The following list emerges from some of the literature in CME:

- active learner participation;
- interaction;

- capacity to develop critical thinking;
- learning from one another;
- exploring perceptions;
- adult learning;
- problem-solving;
- self-directed learning (to an extent);
- exploring different opinions;
- building on previous experience and prior knowledge;
- relevant to practice;
- acquisition of technical skills (but see skills teaching).

   You may have thought of others, but among the characteristics they share is greater personal responsibility for how learners engage with the process. This, in turn, can cause anxiety for a group leader about what might go wrong.

Activity 4.2
Your response may include some of the following:
- lack of participation;
- silence;
- 'difficult' group members;
- loss of control;
- irrelevant discussion;
- learners not learning anything;
- not knowing the answers.

Activity 4.3
There are a number, but a good one might be:
Instructor: OK, who can *tell* me the criteria we are going to use to make our decision as to who will be treated first?

Activity 4.4
People often say that it is the man leaning forward, but in an effective group it could be any one of the others. The facilitator should only lean forward into the group when ready to make an intervention.

Chapter 5 **Teaching skills**

5.1 Learning outcomes

By the end of this chapter, you will be able to demonstrate an understanding of the four-stage approach to skills teaching.

5.2 Introduction

A highly successful approach to teaching skills derives from the work of Gagne[1] and was adapted in the 1980s by the Advanced Trauma Life Support course in their ground breaking programme for managing trauma.[2] Based on behaviourist psychology, skills teaching uses repetition and reinforcement to embed skills in learners so that they do not have to think of the discrete elements of a skill when confronted with the need to act quickly and efficiently. The effective use of skills depends on a complex interrelationship between knowledge and psychomotor ability that we take for granted in those skills that we have already acquired. Those that we have not, however, particularly in adulthood, offer greater challenges.

The ability to develop autonomy, the highest level in psychomotor skills, depends on passing through a number of stages:[3]

- perception;
- guided response;
- mastery;
- autonomy.

In order to explore this process, we take each of these in turn.

Perception

Perception is an awareness of characteristic psychomotor behaviours associated with a skill. This can be consciously and deliberately acquired, or can

How to Teach Continuing Medical Education. By Mike Davis and Kirsty Forrest. Published 2008 by Blackwell Publishing. ISBN: 978-1-4051-5398-0

arise from observation. A child's earliest experience of driving, for example, would come from being driven by a parent or other adult. A child is interested in what is happening but is not trying to learn and the adult is not trying to teach.

Guided response

This arises from a close analysis by the instructor or instructional designer of a given skill. Essentially, a skill is broken down into its component parts and this is far from a straightforward process, involving task analysis in considerable detail. Each sub-skill is taught either separately or in close proximity, and these are combined as a skill. These skills are then themselves combined into the complete repertoire of behaviour associated with the desired behaviour. Learning to drive continues to be a useful analogy:

1 *Skill:* pulling away from the kerb;
2 *Sub-skills:*
  - starting the engine;
  - checking in rear view mirror/wing mirror;
  - depressing clutch;
  - selecting first gear;
  - gentle pressure on the accelerator;
  - easing off pressure on the clutch;
  - handbrake off;
  - turning steering wheel;
  - checking rear view mirror/wing mirror;
  - more pressure on the accelerator;
  - straightening up;
  - changing up to second gear (itself a collection of sub-skills).

ACTIVITY 5.1

Think of a simple psychomotor skill that you use regularly. It need not be a clinical skill. Analyse it in the way demonstrated above. *See end of chapter for response.*

Guided response takes a number of repetitions depending on the complexity of the skill (and the number of contributing sub-skills). After sufficient repetitions, a candidate may be considered to have mastery. This is the point at which, for example, the learner driver successfully passes a driving test. However, the extent to which the learner has, at this point, achieved expertise is less than assured.

Mastery

When I passed my driving test I asked my instructor (from whom I had hired a car for the test) if I could drive home. He was quick to deny my request, arguing that while I had passed my test, I had yet to fully demonstrate autonomy, which is the capacity to think creatively and beyond the boundaries of the instruction and the related test. In other words, I have been trained to pass the test.

This did not mean that I could not drive; rather for some weeks after the test, my driving was characterized by a degree of hesitancy and caution as I became used to (for example) being on my own in the car. In retrospect, it is not possible to identify a moment when I felt that I had absolute control of my actions, but this was the point at which I had achieved the following.

Autonomy

At this point, I can regard myself as an expert and I no longer think of the component skills associated with driving: they are automatic.

Dreyfus and Dreyfus[4] produced a useful analysis of expertise and considered that learners go through stages before acquiring that capacity:

Stage	Characterized by
Novice	Rigid adherence to taught rules or plans Little situational perception No discretionary judgement
Advanced beginner	Guidelines for action based on attributes or aspects Situational perception still limited All attributes and aspects are treated separately and given equal importance
Competent	Coping with multiple actions Now sees actions at least partly in terms of longer-term goals Conscious deliberate planning Standardized and routinized procedures
Proficient	Sees situations holistically rather than in terms of aspects Sees what is most important in a situation Perceives deviations from the normal pattern Decision-making less laboured Uses maxims for guidance, where meaning varies according to the situation
Expert	No longer relies on rules, guidelines or maxims Intuitive grasp of situations based on deep tacit understanding Analytic approaches used only in novel situations or when problems occur Vision of what is possible

The notion of expertise is the same as that explored by Sir John Tooke.[5]

Relationship of skills teaching to learning styles

In some respects, this approach to skills teaching builds on learning style preferences explored earlier in Chapter 1 for:

- visual;
- auditory; and
- kinaesthetic

learners, as follows:

	Nature of demonstration	Who does what	Taxonomy level	Learning style appeal
Stage 1	Real time	Instructor demo	Perception	Predominantly visual
Stage 2	Explanation of the 'what' and 'why'	Instructor demo + instructor commentary	Perception	Visual; auditory (knowledge and comprehension from the cognitive domain)
Stage 3	Learner recall (subject to instructor error-correction and prompt)	Instructor demo + learner commentary	Guided response	Visual and auditory
Stage 4	Psychomotor memory (subject to instructor error-correction and prompt)	Learner performance + learner commentary	Guided response moving towards mastery	Kinaesthetic and auditory

Skills can be taught in this way in groups with up to six members. Beyond this, there would be the potential for some learners to lose interest because of the amount of repetition and redundancy.

The four-stage approach is now explored in more detail, but before doing so, environment and set need attention.

ACTIVITY 5.2

Think about the preparation you would need to undertake in order to teach a skill. *See end of chapter for response.*

The dialogue of a skills station is made up of the four stages, as follows.

Stage 1 – real time demonstration

The real time demonstration was at one time called the 'silent run-through' and this led to the unedifying sight of instructors miming 'Help' (e.g. in Basic Life Support skills training).

In this stage, the instructor wants to show learners the complete skill in the time it takes to do it. So, for example, if the skill is intubation, it is of enormous value to learners to know how quick in practice it should be. It is not carried out silently like a Marcel Marceau mime: you would ask out loud for cricoid pressure or a bougie. However, this is the stage where there is a tendency to anticipate stage 2. This would mean that for endotracheal intubation this could take up to 15 minutes and the student could be under the impression that they can take this long to do it in real life.

The other key issue is that if the instructor were to talk about the components of the skill at this stage, the likelihood is that the learners would look at the instructor's face, rather than his/her hands (Fig. 5.1).

Clearly, this is a *visual* experience.

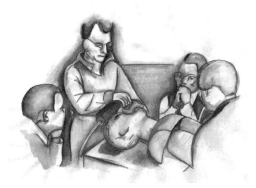

Figure 5.1   A real time demonstration

Stage 2 – instructor demonstration with instructor commentary

At this stage, the instructor repeats the demonstration but, on this occasion, offers explanations as to what is happening and, as importantly, why. Skills do not only depend on psychomotor ability – they do rely on a degree of knowledge, for example in the case of intubation, on learner familiarity with the anatomy of the upper airway and the physiology of respiration; what position the head and neck should be in and how long to attempt intubation. This is also the first opportunity for learners to ask questions of the instructor and possibly to draw on their own and others' personal experiences.

Stage 3 – instructor demonstration and learner commentary

This important third stage has three possible processes:

1 The instructor takes the lead and the learner *describes* what is happening.
2 The instructor *follows* the learner's instructions.
3 A mixture of both of these.

In the case of the first of these, the learner may still be uncertain and the additional repetition with the instructor taking the lead offers another round of reinforcement.

In the second case, the learner appears confident and assured and can safely lead the instructor in undertaking the skill.

In the final case, the learner begins to lead the instructor but becomes hesitant and so the instructor takes the lead until the learner regains confidence.

In all three cases, it is the instructor's responsibility to correct error at this stage: other, perhaps less confident, learners are still acting as observers and they need to see identical and accurate performances of the skill each time it is demonstrated.

As with stage 2, this stage stimulates the visual and auditory learner.

Stage 4 – learner demonstration with learner commentary

At this stage, learners take it in turns to demonstrate the skill while at the same time providing a commentary about what they are doing. The role of the instructor is to listen and watch carefully and to correct any errors.

The process described above is of particular value in a classroom or clinical skills laboratory and it is true that it lends itself well to the teaching of discrete skills that take seconds or minutes rather than hours to complete. However, complex multifaceted tasks can be disaggregated to a series of sub-skills which can be taught discretely and then reassembled as a complete procedure.

This approach to instruction can teach quite complex skills as long as they are relevant to learners' needs and to their cognitive understanding gained elsewhere. It is expected that the learning design of the course as a whole would reflect the learners' need for the skill. There is considerable evidence that skills, if not practiced, decay after a relatively short period of time.

The behaviour that is being taught in skills teaching is the capacity for automatic responses: there is no time to disaggregate the steps and there is some evidence to suggest that if you think too hard about the steps that make up a skill, you are likely to perform these suboptimally. Both driving and walking down stairs are examples of this, although they should not be tried at home.

Four-stage teaching approach over time

The way in which skills teaching has been described in this chapter so far is based on the assumption that the skill is going to be taught within a discrete period of time in a discrete location. However, it is possible by using video recordings of stages 1 and 2 to prepare learners for the more hands-on experiences in a clinical skills workshop. Advanced Paediatric Life Support (APLS) skills are now taught this way in the APLS Virtual Learning Environment.[6]

Other approaches to skills teaching

Simulator training

Most surgeons will now be trained and assessed in simulators. Advances in technology mean that there are very lifelike simulators for keyhole surgery, endoscopies and full-scale high fidelity resuscitations. Many include software so that the simulator's reactions depend on the trainee's actions. There are many advantages to simulator training. The most obvious is that students can practice as often as they like and whenever they want (within reason) without harming a patient. Continual improvement with appropriate feedback is a form of deliberate practice. In the 1970s, scientists wanted to find out how long it took to become an expert in a particular field and observed master chess and piano players; the figure of 10,000 hours or 10 years of practice evolved.[7] Ericsson took this further and said to be an expert you had to be able reproduce superior performance and to do this took deliberate practice.[8]

Deliberate practice may seem a strange use of words; however, it emphasizes that you need appropriate feedback to improve. All aspects of our professional life need this to improve. Conference participants were discussing the importance of encouraging experienced academics to develop their teaching. One rose to say: 'some say they have 20 years' experience of teaching – but in reality they have only one; they have simply repeated it each of the following 19 years' (attributed to Lewis Elton, Honorary Professor of Higher Education, University College London).

Simulator training is a less threatening educational environment than real life. There is a full range of fidelities available; however, there is mounting evidence that without the proper educational input (e.g. providing good feedback) they are at best a waste of money.

The Best Evidence Medical Education collaboration (BEME Systematic Review)[9] concluded that the following need to feature in effective skills teaching using simulators:
- feedback;
- practice;
- validity;
- curriculum integration;
- outcomes defined;
- variety of conditions;
- range of difficulty;
- controlled setting.

Skills teaching in the workplace

While the four-stage technique works well for courses, it sometimes does not easily translate into the workplace and may have to be modified. During clinical practice there can be a conflict of interest with a real patient in front of you and a student who wants to learn a skill. It may not be possible to use the teaching opportunities because of other priorities – the patient may be so sick that the consultant may not deem it appropriate to supervise while also managing the patient. Success of the technique may be so crucial that the consultant may not wish the chances of success to be jeopardized by the trainee.

The modular approach to 'chunking' of the skill will still work. However, there are other stages prior to the one to be taught and learnt, and while they are closely related, they belong to the area of attitudinal rather than psychomotor skills:
- Is the skill the right decision at that time for that patient?
- Has the trainee explained the procedure to the patient?

The Direct Observation of Procedural Skills (DOPS) shows other aspects of a procedural skill for the purposes of work-based assessment.

DOPS assessment criteria:
1 demonstrates understanding of anatomy, indications for procedure and technique;
2 obtains informed consent;
3 demonstrates appropriate preparation preprocedure;
4 appropriate analgesia or safe sedation;
5 technical ability;
6 aseptic technique;
7 seeks help where appropriate;
8 postprocedure management;

9 communication skills;

10 consideration of patient/professionalism;

11 overall ability to perform procedure (global score).

All this emphasizes that a practical procedure is more than a technical skill. This can be put simply: the measures of success of a practical procedure are:

- a correct decision to undertake the procedure;
- proper technical performance of the procedure;
- the correct outcome.

Good preplanning is essential to teaching a skill. There must be agreement on a technique (e.g. teaching a lumber puncture), which approach, how many attempts allowed, key words or phrases to indicate that you are going to take over from the trainee. For example, 'Good, now that you have completed your part of the procedure I shall begin mine.' This can be done with the four-handed technique (both of you with gloves on – trainer directing the trainee hands-on.)

The other classic is the 'magic gloves' technique. When a trainee looks as if they are struggling to perform a task the guarantee is that when you, the trainer, decide to take over and put on the sterile procedural gloves, the trainee miraculously is able to do what they were previously struggling to do. Obviously, in these circumstances, the trainer retains responsibility for the safe completion of the skill.

ACTIVITY 5.3

From your own experience of learning a new skill, were you properly supervised? What features made supervision good or poor? *See end of chapter for response.*

The learning curve

Technical skills can be predicted and some learners are better than others. The learning curve is only associated with poor outcomes when trainees are unsupervised. The learning curve depends on the frequency of the encounter, the quality of encounter, the quality of feedback but not necessarily the complexity of the task.

It is useful to compare skills acquisition to the UK driving test. After passing your driving test, the learning curve is not yet complete, but the driver is now considered able to progress along that curve without any further direct supervision (Fig. 5.2).

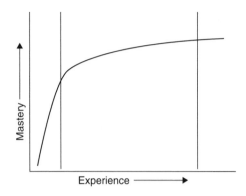

Figure 5.2 A learning curve

Circle of failure

Some people are poor at performing new skills. This can be for a number of reasons:

- procedural inertia;
- dexterity decay;
- struggle or failure;
- loss of confidence.

The reason that some struggle to acquire skills can be inherent to the person (e.g. a trait ability or lack of coordination). However, this is rare and more often than not they have actually been taught the wrong way, had improper reinforcement and think they are doing it well or have not seen the skill performed properly in the first place. Sometimes, what develops is a circle of failure which we all have probably experienced. A bad experience is associated with that skill, either rightly or wrongly, and from then on a self-perpetuating circle of apprehension and fear develops around the skill. First of avoidance and therefore less exposure to the skill and then when performing the skill fear can cause performance degradation and the circle continues. The only way to address this is to admit it is happening and start from the beginning again with the four-stage technique, with a friendly competent colleague.

In conclusion, there is a wide range of performance demonstrable with any practical skill, and with rapid improvement in the learning curve in first 20–30 cases. There is generally a consistent improvement thereafter but only with deliberate practice. Practice is essential to prevent skill decay and some people will learn faster than others.

References

1 Gagne R. *The Conditions of Learning* (4th edn.) 1985. Holt, Rinehart & Winston, New York.

2 American College of Surgeons Committee on Trauma. *Advanced Trauma Life Support for Doctors* (7th edn.) 2004. American College of Surgeons, Chicago.

3 Mackway-Jones K, Walker M. *Pocket Guide to Teaching for Medical Instructors.* 1999. BMJ Books, London.

4 Dreyfus H, Dreyfus S. *Mind over Machine: The Power of Human Intuition and Expertise in the Era of the Computer.* 1986. Basil Blackwell, Oxford.

5 Tooke J. *Aspiring to Excellence: Findings and Recommendations of the Independent Inquiry into Modernising Medical Careers.* 2007. Aldridge Press, Chiswick.

6 http://www.alsg.org/index.php?id=26. Accessed 3 February 2008.

7 Simon HA, Chase RA. Skill in chess. *American Scientist* 1973;**61**:394–403.

8 Ericsson KA. Deliberate practice and the acquisition and maintenance of expert performance in medicine and related domains. *Academic Medicine* 2004;**79**: S70–S81.

9 Issenberg S, McGaghie W, Petrusa E, Gordon D, Scalese R. Features and uses of high-fidelity medical simulations that lead to effective learning: a BEME systematic review. *Medical Teacher* 2005;**27**:10–28.

Responses to activities

Activity 5.1
You should include sufficient detail to enable a novice to recognize each of the discrete tasks.

Activity 5.2
You would need to pay attention to:
• *Environment* (heat, light, etc.)
• *Visibility:* Is there room for everyone to be able to see?
• *Equipment:* Is it there? Does it work?
• *Distractions:* Are there other groups close by? Is there superfluous equipment lying around?
• *Introductions:* Do they know who you are? Do you know who they are?

Activity 5.3
Poor: being out of your depth, too high expectations, unclear of task.
Good: reverse of above.

Chapter 6 **Role play and simulated scenarios**

6.1 Learning outcomes

By the end of this chapter you should be able to demonstrate an understanding of:
- the aims of role play and simulated scenarios;
- how to facilitate role plays and simulated scenarios.

6.2 Introduction

Both role play and simulation at first sight belong to a drama tradition: one based on 'let's pretend …' or the notion of 'the willing suspension of disbelief', and while it is true that both contain elements of this tradition, they are both firmly embedded in reality. The perception of *play* can, in fact, run counter to a facilitator's intentions if the activity is not taken seriously. This combined with learners' anxiety about role play can prevent learners from getting full value from the experience unless it is facilitated with confidence and commitment.[1] This will be explored later in the chapter.

Before exploring any further, it is necessary to characterize role play and to examine how it fits into a simulation.

Definition: role play

The key components of a role play is that the learner speaks as:
- a version of themselves in a familiar situation;
- a version of themselves in a novel situation;
- another person in a familiar situation;
- another person in a novel situation;

all within either familiar or novel contexts.

How to Teach Continuing Medical Education. By Mike Davis and Kirsty Forrest. Published 2008 by Blackwell Publishing. ISBN: 978-1-4051-5398-0

As van Ments put it:[2]

Role-play is the name given to one particular type of simulation that focuses attention on the interaction of people with one another. It emphasizes the functions performed by different people under various circumstances.

The role player needs some contextual, biographical and perceptual information to use as a basis for the interaction but a key characteristic of role play is that, in general, there is no predetermined outcome.

Role plays fall into five typical types:[3]

1 *Improvization:* learners use their own responses and actions in a given situation; in other words, they behave as themselves but in novel (to them) context. For example, 'You are in the bar at the theatre when an old man nearby clutches his chest and falls to the floor.'

2 *Structured:* learners are given a role to play with clear instructions on how this should be performed. For example, 'You are a nervous junior doctor confronted with a febrile child and her somewhat hysterical mother.'

3 *Reverse role play:* where learners play a role other than their normal one to gain insight into the thoughts, attitudes and behaviours of others. For example, the learner might play a mother being informed about serious illness in her baby.

4 *Exaggerated role play:* overdeveloping the features of a character to make a particular point. For example, an (over) aggressive relative receiving bad news.

5 *Prepared improvization:* as with improvization but following a discussion as to the nature of the roles, specific episodes and a predetermined outcome.

Whatever approach is employed, there are a number of essential ingredients of a role play session if it is going to have any significant impact on learners. The role play itself (i.e. the episode when one or more learners acts out the scenario) followed by observation, reflection and conceptualization, leading to an exploration of other possible behaviours that may produce better outcomes is a reminder of the experiential learning cycle explored in Chapter 1 and realized, in this description, rather differently, as follows:[1]

Kolb & Fry (1975)[4] describe four learning environments in their theory of experiential learning: affectively oriented (feeling), symbolically oriented (thinking), perceptually oriented (watching), behaviourally oriented (doing). Within each environment there are two tasks. First, 'grasping' which consists of concrete experiences and abstract conceptualization. Second, 'transforming' which consists of reflection and action. Learning is enhanced when learners are encouraged to use all four environments. Structured role-play with feedback enables learners to complete both tasks in each of the four environments.

The key, therefore, to the educational benefit of role play is an opportunity to experiment with interaction without the attendant risks associated with interaction with real patients and their relatives. Habitual behaviour can be tested and feedback can be sought and if necessary, alternatives can be suggested and tested. The importance of observation, reflection, conceptualization and experimentation cannot be underemphasized.

Running a role play

There are some particular issues that need to be taken into consideration when preparing for, and running a role play. While the usual attention has to be paid to the environment, it is also important to attend to some different conditions. These include the following.

Need for privacy

Role players almost always feel somewhat vulnerable so you have to ensure that their work is not overlooked by people beyond the immediate group. This has to be accommodated when planning an event that involves role play.

Layout

Help create an appropriate environment, taking into consideration:
- placement of chairs and other furniture (e.g. a desk for the 'doctor' to take notes);
- a suitable place for observers – not too close; avoiding obvious sight lines;
- a place for the facilitator: you do not want to hover over the group.

Briefing

Each briefing will be in two parts: general information which will be shared by all role players, and specific information for the individual roles. The briefings have to be concise and unambiguous and contain enough information for the role players to engage with one another. They should be told that the can be creative (i.e. invent detail) in the absence of given information, but that it must be credible and consistent. They should be told that the facilitator will manage time boundaries and bring the role play to an end.

Even though a role play is not *real*, it does need to be *realistic* and this also needs thought. Where the facililitator can ensure some feasibility, however, is by ensuring that individuals are given roles they could reasonably be expected to enact: for example, an foundation doctor in Emergency

Medicine might struggle to role play a consultant paediatrician discussing possible child abuse with parents.

The role play

The role play itself should be designed to enable the role players time to deal with all of the issues for consideration and the role of the facilitator is to listen very carefully and not to intervene, by word or gesture, or influence the process in any way. For purposes of post role play debrief and discussion, it may be worthwhile taking notes.

The debrief

In many respects, the post role play discussion is where learning can be maximized for all participants, including observers. Learner and instructor critiquing has been seen in a number of contexts as being the way in which this should occur and approaches to this are explored in a number of places, including Bullock et al.[3] During this time, learners should be encouraged to explore thoughts and feelings and to identify problematic and challenging moments. As far as is possible, from memories of what is after all an ephemeral event, comments and discussion should be based on evidence – what people said, and how they said it. A shared exploration of this can be a powerful learning experience for role players and observers.

Role play has a strong emotional component and participants need to be enabled to return to normal, particularly if they have been dealing with issues that could resonate powerfully with their own experience. This issue is important for all participants, even for doctors role playing 'doctors' because they will not necessarily be functioning within their own comfort zone in the role play and may not have performed as well as they would expect of themselves. Acknowledging this allows role players to own up to error *in role*, rather than feeling defensive about their 'own' performance.

In order to help role players to return to 'real life', ask individual role players to say a little bit about themselves. For example: 'OK John, what are you planning for the weekend?' This will enable John to free himself of the roles he has just undertaken.

Running a simulation

Jones explores the difficulty of reaching an adequate definition of simulations:[5]

> In my first book I criticized existing definitions and expressed a preference for descriptions. But I added, 'If a short definition is really necessary, perhaps it might be "Simulations are reality"'. In my second

book I devised the following definition of an educational simulation: 'Reality of function in a simulated and structured environment' ...
Today I might ask for a little more space, and say something like: 'A simulation in education is an untaught event in which sufficient information is provided to allow the participants to achieve reality of function in a simulated environment.'

Simulations can be thought of as role plays with equipment. They have the capacity to allow learners to integrate their learning from other contexts: reading, lectures, skills stations and workshops. In something approaching real time, learners can interact within a context, including other health specialists acting as assistants and with instructors who provide clinical and other information to prompt learners as to the correct way in which to assess a patient and to make decisions in a way that is, as far as possible, true to life. Kneebone identifies criteria for evaluating simulations:[6]

1 simulations should allow for sustained and deliberate practice in a safe environment and that simulations ensure skills are consolidated and aligned with other curricula activity;
2 simulations should provide access to expert tutors who are available only when needed;
3 simulations should map on to real life clinical experience;
4 simulation-based learning should provide a supportive, motivational and learner-centred environment.

At the heart of simulation teaching is a role play in which a learner tries to replicate behaviour mastered in previous teaching episodes. The environment for a simulation is, however, considerably more complex, involving equipment, assistants and decisions (for the organizer) about manikins or actors.

Equipment will depend entirely on the nature of the scenario – an outline of an hypothesized chain of events – being offered. Clearly, there will be a difference between what you need for a paediatric resuscitation in an emergency department and what you would be looking for in a critical care area. The best way to determine what you need is to 'walk through' the scenario. This will allow you also to make a number of decisions about what is missing. This process can also alert you to any other uncertainties or ambiguities that are present in the scenario story.

ACTIVITY 6.1

You have obtained a Simman™ manikin and you think it would be a good way to teach the trainees on how to deal with critical incidents.
How would you start to prepare? *See end of chapter for response.*

An aside about manikins, high-fidelity simulators and actors
The purpose of simulation is to provide opportunities for health professionals to learn sometimes complex procedures away from actual patients,
who, for fairly obvious reasons cannot be seen as an arena for trying out
new skills.

As Small writes:[7]

> First and foremost, this type of training uncouples patient injury
> from learning and sends a message to all stakeholders including
> the public that patients are not a commodity for training. Second,
> learning opportunities can be custom-designed to maximize the
> training process for teachers and learners. Learning theory has shown
> that trainees learn differently, at different rates, have different needs,
> and benefit most from experiential methods that enable the most
> efficient 'transfer' from practice to operations. Third, simulation
> fosters social justice, in that the great majority of novice training
> occurs at academic medical centers where vulnerable inner city
> populations receive care. Fourth, simulation techniques are ideally
> adapted to learning error management skills. Rich, immediate
> feedback can be provided while allowing tasks and events to unfold
> to the degree necessary to accomplish learning objectives. In actual,
> operational environments, dangerous errors must be corrected at
> once, often by those with the most experience, and little time is
> available for post-event debriefing. Nuanced data from real events
> is often not captured, and the ability to replay the experience is
> impossible.

The opportunity for debrief is a key component of the simulated experience as this is where learning can be maximized. Many simulator centres
have the ability to video the experience through a one-way mirror and this
provides the opportunity for the participants to replay and analyse their
own performance.

Non-technical skills
Non-technical skills include decision-making, situation awareness and team
working. The ability to diagnose and treat the right patient at the right time
is what all medical teachers are aiming for from their students. The development of non-technical skill teaching in general has been led by the aviation
industry. In the 1970s, it was discovered that many air disasters were the
result of lack of communication and poor team working and not because
of hardware failure or lack of flying skills. The adoption of human factors
training into medicine has been driven by patient safety and anaesthesia has

been one speciality that has embraced the training (maybe because of the perceived similarities to flying).[8]

With simulated scenarios, the trainer can explore trainees' non-technical skills. By avoiding the most obvious and sometimes confrontational question: 'Why did you do that?' post experience discussion can be used to explore clinical reasoning.

Imagine, the activity above had been to teach trainees about the diagnosis and treatment of anaphylaxis on the Simman™. During the replay of the scenario, the video could be stopped and questions asked that help to explore situational awareness, such as:

- 'What data were you considering to arrive at the conclusion of anaphylaxis?'
- 'What else did you want to know in order to make the decision and how did that help decide?'
- 'What made you go for that option?'
- 'Which bit of information on the monitor was out of keeping with the rest?'

More questions can be asked to explore decision-making:

- 'What else could you have done to treat anaphylaxis?'
- 'Did you think you made the right decision?'
- 'Did the treatment work as you expected?'
- 'Would you do the same next time?'

This form of teaching is thought to accelerate the learning of tacit knowledge and in this age of reduced exposure to real life experiences is of vital importance. Fletcher *et al.*[9] have developed a behavioural marking system for these skills providing a more formal way to train and assess participants.

6.3 Conclusions and learning

Role play and scenario teaching differ from other teaching modalities in the way in which, if successful, they relate directly to practice. They utilize skills, knowledge and affect in order to enable learners to explore a simulation of their real world.

As an instructor, you should aspire to make the simulations as lifelike as necessary to maximize the learning experience for all participants.

References

1 Nestel D, Tierney T. Role-play for medical students learning about communication: Guidelines for maximising benefits. *BMC Medical Education.* 2007;7:3 [doi:10.1186/1472-6920-7-3].

2 van Ments M. *The Effective Use of Role Play: A Handbook for Teachers & Trainers.* 1983. Kogan Page, London.

3 Bullock I, Davis M, Lockey A, Mackway-Jones K. (eds.) *Pocket Guide to Teaching for Medical Educators* (2nd edn). 2008. Blackwell, Oxford.

4 Kolb D, Fry R. Toward an applied theory of experiential learning. In Cooper C. (ed.) *Theories of Group Process.* 1975. John Wiley, London.

5 Jones K. *Designing Your Own Simulations.* 1985. Methuen, London.

6 Kneebone R. Evaluating clinical simulations for learning procedural skills: A theory-based approach. *Academic Medicine* 2005;**80**:549–553.

7 Small S. Thoughts on patient safety education and the role of simulation. *Virtual Mentor* 2004;**6**:3 [http://virtualmentor.ama-assn.org/2004/03/medu1-0403.html accessed on 26 October 2007].

8 Gaba D. Anaesthesiology as a model for patient safety in health care. *BMJ* 2000;**320**:785–788.

9 Fletcher G, Flin R, McGeorge P, Glavin R, Maran N, Patey R. Rating non-technical skills: Developing a behavioural marker system for use in anaesthesia. *Cognition, Technology & Work* 2004;**6**:165–171.

Response to activity

Activity 6.1

Be very specific about your educational goals – sometimes it is very easy to get carried away with the technology and forget the reason that you are there. Once you have set out your aims and objectives, be very specific about your scenarios. It is helpful to write these down as a flow diagrams as this is often what the computer programs for the manikins look like.

Try to anticipate student replies; think outside the box as some replies or actions can be very surprising and have an appropriate reply or action from the manikin ready. Practice on the manikin running through the scenario – this is when you find that the physical signs of the manikin that you expected sometimes are not present and you will have to adjust the scenario to maintain realism. You will be 'walking through' the scenario, gathering kit and turning the environment into a realistic set. Enrol the help of a colleague: often you need one person to run the scenario (and manikin) and the other to actually assess the trainee, especially when looking at non-technical skills.

Chapter 7 **Clinical teaching**

There should be no teaching without the patient for a text and the best teaching is often that taught by the patient himself. (Osler)[1]

7.1 Learning outcomes

By the end of this chapter, you will be able to demonstrate an understanding of effective approaches to clinical teaching.

7.2 Introduction

Clinical teaching has many benefits over more formal teaching episodes as it is patient rather than disease orientated. Interaction between patients and doctors can demonstrate a positive attitude towards learning through active participation rather than passive observation. Learners are exposed to a model of practice that they can go on to apply to their own interactions with patients. The integration of clinical medicine with basic sciences is shown on real patients and there is generally an emphasis on the teaching of applied problem-solving – as most of medicine is good detective work. Teaching in clinical settings provides good role models of interpersonal relationships with patients and colleagues for the learners.

Clinical teaching brings together six domains of knowledge,[2] as follows:[3]

> Clinical knowledge of medicine, of patients, and the context of practice; and educational knowledge of learners, general principles of teaching and case based teaching scripts.

and as such is congruent with the model of learning embodied by situated cognition explored in Chapter 1.

How to Teach Continuing Medical Education. By Mike Davis and Kirsty Forrest. Published 2008 by Blackwell Publishing. ISBN: 978-1-4051-5398-0

7.3 The challenges of clinical teaching

There are challenges with clinical teaching, often seen as separate from the actual job of practicing medicine. There can be a perceived conflict of interest for clinicians, with time for teaching considered separate from that for caring for patients. There is also an increase in competing demands of other roles in management, administration and research. There is a general lack of reward and recognition for this type of teaching within the health service. In addition, with the increasing numbers of students and decreasing numbers of inpatients (with the move to community-based care), the opportunities for this type of teaching are decreasing. The clinical environment is not always conducive for teaching and learning, with space often at a premium.

A workshop recently held with clinical teachers and trainees looked at addressing issues around clinical teaching. The trainees raised the following points as bad examples of clinical teaching:
- lack of objectives given;
- teaching pitched at wrong level;
- passive observation rather than active participation;
- inadequate supervision;
- no feedback provided;
- teaching by humiliation still occurs;
- teachers being unaware of where the subject sits with the rest of the curriculum.

The points raised generally revolve around lack of preparation on the part of the teacher. However, as explored elsewhere in this book, there are certain things that a medical educator can do to improve the learning experience.

7.4 Characteristics of a good clinical teacher

Many medics have memories of the Sir Lancelot Spratt moments on teaching ward rounds. Here is a reminder:[4]

Sir Lancelot, an eminent abdominal surgeon, happens to be on a ward round with a huge entourage of nurses, understudies and medical students. The hapless patient has need of a cholecystectomy for gallstones, and the team are all discussing the size of the incision necessary to carry out this procedure. When the medical student suggests a rather conservative-size cut, Sir Lancelot roars, 'Don't be stupid boy!' and gestures an incision with his pencil several inches long across the patient's hypochondrium. When the patient shrieks and starts to question this, Sir Lancelot shouts 'Shut up man! This is nothing to do with you!'

All of these characteristics can be developed by clinical teachers and what follows are a number of models that may be helpful.

One minute preceptor

Clinical teachers can adopt different roles in a clinical setting: that of expert consultant, joint problem-solver, didactic teacher or, where appropriate, the one minute preceptor (OMP). This approach was developed in the USA in 1992 as the 'five step microskills model of clinical teaching' and is in marked contrast to the more traditional bedside approach where the focus is on diagnosing the patient's problem rather than the learner's needs.

The OMP model focuses the teaching encounter on the learner's reasoning while simultaneously gathering the necessary components of the history and physical exam. This is similar to asking open ended questions of patients to gather the history, rather than jumping right into direct questioning. This model allows the preceptor to assess the learner's knowledge and reasoning, and provide key messages for learning.

Key steps of the OMP model, along with selected suggested phrases to use, include:

- Get a commitment from the learner about the need to identify the nature of the problem: 'What do you think is going on with the patient?'
- Probe for underlying reasoning: 'What were the major findings that lead you to this diagnosis or decision? What else did you consider? What other information might you need?'
- Teach general rules (key teaching points).
- Provide positive feedback.
- Correct errors in reasoning.

An example of OMP

The 'sick patient'. In the medical admissions unit, a junior doctor (conscientious but somewhat insecure about her knowledge and skill) presents the following case to you:

> I have just finished admitting a 35-year-old man. He has been complaining of general body pain for a few days. He also complains of being short of breath and a productive cough. He denies any

blood in the sputum. He is a non-smoker and is not a bird keeper. On physical examination, he looks unwell, his vital signs are heart rate 100 beats/min, blood pressure 110/70 mmHg, respiratory rate 18 breaths/min and his temperature is 38.5°C. I tried to listen to his chest but was unsure what I heard. Also, I would like to do a blood gas but last time I couldn't manage that. I was unsure what to do next as he seems very unwell.

(Preceptor as expert consultant: 'Get on with doing the ABCs and start antibiotics.')

Preceptor: 'What do you think is his problem?' (Skill 1: Getting a commitment.)

Student: 'I am concerned that he might be septic.'

Preceptor: 'What makes you think he might be septic?' (Skill 2: Probe for underlying reasoning.)

Student: 'He has abnormal vital signs, with a productive cough; he may have a chest infection.'

Preceptor: 'Yes the vital signs are abnormal. We need to make sure that we have done the ABCs properly first. The chest infection is a logical possibility but we don't have adequate information to confirm the diagnosis. We need a more complete physical examination, particularly of the respiratory system and a chest X-ray. Do you want me to model how to treat this patient or would you like me to observe you do them?' (Skills 3: Teach general rules.)

Student: 'I would really appreciate you observing me please.'

Preceptor: 'OK. Let's go and see the patient together.'

The ABCs are performed on the patient. The student proceeds to examine the patient's chest. Here the preceptor may want to change the role to that of a didactic teacher or problem-solver, depending on the student's performance.

Preceptor: 'How did you think you did on that chest examination?'

Student: 'Not as well as I would have liked.'

Teacher: 'What went well?'

Student: 'This time I could hear some added sounds at the left base, where as before I heard nothing.'

Teacher: 'You positioned the patient appropriately for the examination.' (Skill 4: Provide positive feedback.) 'I would recommend that next time you fully expose the patient as this will make it a lot easier to listen to the chest.' (Skill 5: Correct errors in reasoning.)

The OMP has been shown to be an effective method for teaching because of its focus on students' deeper thinking – exploring processes rather than superficial factual knowledge. While there might be legitimate concerns about how long this exploration make take, studies have shown that the use of time is more efficient, enabling the clinician to manage patient care information while at the same time supporting students' knowledge and understanding.[7]

Teaching one-to-one

Teaching one-to-one (TONTO) can be a luxury for a busy clinician. However, operating theatres and general practice, by virtue of space constraints, are settings where TONTO is often a necessity.

There are many advantages of TONTO for both the learner and the teacher:

- no competing demands of other learners and the teacher can pitch material at the appropriate level;
- provides the opportunity to explore the trainee's understanding of material at a deeper level than in a group setting;
- feedback can be more timely and specific.

Disadvantages include:

- there can be blurring of roles for the clinician between teacher, mentor, counsellor and friend;
- student and teacher personality differences can be a complicating factor;
- lack of social learning support from fellow learners.

The effective application of TONTO demands particular attention to the nature of the relationship between the teacher and taught, something Lyon[8] described as 'sizing up'. This mutual process can lead to feelings of trust and legitimacy which in turn validates the learner's presence as a legitimate peripheral participant[5] in the community of practice.

Ward rounds

The typical ward round is seen as an important part of patient care and not necessarily a teaching opportunity. However, forethought and a little planning can provide a rich learning environment. The relationships between nursing staff, patients and doctors are presented to learners, along with the decision-making process.

Running a teaching ward round

There are a number of preconditions that enable a ward round to become a successful learning opportunity:

1 Liaise with nursing staff:
  - If at all possible, have a nurse accompany the ward round. This helps to introduce the trainees to a team approach of medical care.

2 Set some boundaries with trainees before the round:
   - Remind the trainees that words such as cancer can be frightening to patients.
3 Put the patient at ease:
   - introduce yourself and your team to the patient;
   - let the patient know that there will be diseases and diagnoses mentioned that do not apply to them;
   - reassure the patient that he/she is free to ask questions and make comments;
   - use the patient's name and involve them in discussion;
   - emphasize the patient's importance in his/her role as a teacher.
4 Involve the students and observe them in action:
   - this can range from talking to a patient, checking physical signs, presenting the case history, answering questions from you, other students and the patient;
   - rotate the questions and activities;
   - make sure all students have been involved in some activities at least once.
5 Give immediate feedback about performance.
6 Be honest – say 'I don't know' if you truly do not know but offer ways of finding out.
7 Teach professionalism – respect the patient, their privacy and wishes.
8 Debriefing after the round:
   - see if experience gained can be incorporated into existing knowledge and experience;
   - explore any unanswered questions.
9 Give homework to trainees to look up for next time you meet.
10 Keep the ward round to a reasonable length.

A colleague mentioned that she did not like having trainees on her ward round. They slowed her down and they could not be trusted to give the same high standard of care that she delivered – after all she was the consultant. We discussed this and developed plans for future ward rounds that would help educate as well as 'get the work done' of caring for patients:

- assigning each trainee roles for the day – scribe, prescriber, examiner and history-taker, which can be rotated over the week;
- dividing the team in two, with each taking opposite ends of the ward and meeting in the middle to discuss all patients;
- 'teaching' on only 2–3 patients for that day, explaining this to the trainees and the patients;
- have an 'investigation of the day' (e.g. ECGs, X-rays or blood results) that teaching will be concentrated on.

Patient centred medical education

All the above models of learning are based on consultant led or student centred approaches. These models have the patient as an almost peripheral entity to the relationship between teacher/knowledge giver and the student. Bleakley and Bligh has postulated that by putting the patient at the centre of the relationship, students can learn about gaps in their knowledge instead of role modelling behaviour from consultants or deciding for themselves what is missing. As they write:[9]

> Focussing medical education on the patient–student dialogue, with the doctor as expert support, offers the conditions of possibility for a co-production of knowledge where the student reads the patient as text in a more holistic manner, within which a specific clinical narrative is embedded.

The patient becomes the educator and the consultant a facilitator. While this has been a popular current model, much of the teaching has concentrated on communication training and the development of empathy and reflection and not on developing a true relationship with patients. In addition, other relationships in the health care system need to be modelled to show the true symbiosis that exists.[10]

These models naturally lend themselves to smaller institutions where the community-based aspects of the learning can be brought to the fore.

7.5 Opportunistic teaching

All of the foregoing approaches to clinical teaching share the characteristic of being opportunistic and clinical teaching has been indelibly linked with opportunistic teaching or teaching on the run. Opportunistic learning episodes occur frequently within clinical settings, but these are not always used to their full potential. Opportunistic teaching is often misinterpreted by both students and teachers as not requiring preparation or forethought but, as with all teaching, this not true. When planning clinical teaching the following questions should be asked:

- How long will the students be with you?
- What have the students done before?
- What will the students do next?
- What do the students expect to happen?
- What are the intended learning outcomes of this placement?
- How will the students be assessed?
- Who else is involved in teaching and learning at this point?
- What are your expectations of them?

- Where can teaching take place?
- Who else might be involved in teaching?
- What special resources can you offer?

The range of teaching techniques and methodologies that need to be employed in each setting is varied but all follow the basic principles described below.

ACTIVITY 7.2

You are a consultant cardiologist in a teaching hospital. The coronary care unit is busy and you think there are many learning opportunities available. The trainees appear disinterested and not motivated on the ward rounds. What could you do? *See end of chapter for response.*

Clinical teachers often have little idea about their students' learning needs and tend to focus on knowledge objectives that could be met by other means such as text books. There should be a shift from what clinicians want to teach to what trainees need to learn: changing the educational methodology from a teacher centred to a learner centred approach. Adults like to have an input into their learning.

Knowing the learners

Although clinical teachers may be actively teaching, there is a risk that our current teaching practices encourage passivity and dependence in our learners by focusing on facts rather than problem-solving. Self-directed learning has huge potential educational value but in order to motivate and engage students in it, we have to find ways to make it more enjoyable and clinically relevant.

Learners will travel along the continuum of dependency of learning and also may regress depending on circumstances. As trainees progress, there is a move from being dependent, to being interested and to being self-directed. Teaching styles need to take into account junior doctors' prior knowledge and their stage of learning. Expecting busy junior doctors to define their own needs, or presenting a mini-lecture to a mature and enquiring registrar, will demotivate both. Nevertheless, a degree of mismatch can challenge a learner and be a good thing. Shifting teaching styles from didactic to delegating, moves the workload away from us and makes teaching and learning more fun. On the other hand, we all like to learn in different ways at different times and sometimes a didactic presentation is all we want. As teachers, we need to be flexible to suit the learners and the circumstances.

Challenges

Not all opportunities that arise in the clinical setting are naturally good teaching or learning moments. You could have had a bad night on call or the case maybe particularly challenging and you cannot perform as a teacher to the best of your ability. The best approach is to be realistic, to acknowledge that it is sometimes impossible to deliver high quality teaching in all clinical situations. In these circumstances, you need to negotiate with students and explain why. Enrolling colleagues to help with teaching can be appropriate at these times. Our understanding of these challenges arises from the work of Maslow, outlined in Chapter 1. The physiological needs have to be met if learning is going to take place, and this applies as much to you as instructor as it does to your trainees who may not be used to going without lunch or being on their feet for 8 hours.

7.6 Conclusions

Clinical teaching is an important aspect for continuing medical education. Fortunately, the mainstay for this type of teaching is the same as for all educational episodes: maintaining a clear vision of your teaching outcomes, knowing your audience and knowing your material.

References

1 Bliss M. *William Osler: A Life in Medicine.* 1999. Oxford University Press, New York.
2 Irby, D.M. What clinical teachers in medicine need to know. *Academic Medicine* 1994;69(5):333–342.
3 Harris I. Qualitative methods. In Norman G, van der Vleuten C, Newble D. (eds.) *International Handbook of Research in Medical Education: Part 1.* 2002. Kluwer.
4 Charlton R. (ed.) *Learning to Consult.* 2007. Radcliffe Publishing, Oxford.
5 Lave J, Wenger, E. *Situated Learning: Legitimate Peripheral Participation.* 1991. Cambridge University Press, Cambridge.
6 Launer J. *Supervision, Mentoring and Coaching: One-to-One Learning Encounters in Medical Education.* 2006. ASME, Edinburgh: p. 4.
7 Aagaard E, Teherani A, Irby D. Effectiveness of the one-minute preceptor model for diagnosing the patient and the learner: Proof of concept. *Academic Medicine* 2004;**79**:42–49.
8 Lyon P. A model of teaching and learning in the operating theatre. *Medical Education* 2004;**38**:1278–1287.
9 Bleakley A, Bligh J. Students learning from patients: Let's get real in medical education. *Advances in Health Science Education* [http://www.springer.com accessed on 31 October2006]

10 Prideaux D, Worley P, Bligh J. Symbiosis: A new model for medical education. *The Clinical Teacher* 2007;**4**:209–212.

11 Rushworth B. Teaching medical students: The student's perspective. *The Clinical Teacher* 2004;**1**:46–48.

Responses to activities

Activity 7.1

You may have thought about some of these:

- enthusiastic about teaching;
- interested in the well-being of students;
- capacity for dialogue (as opposed to teacherly monologue);
- well prepared;
- teaching in the context of real medical problems;
- capacity to be tentative;
- organized;
- being prepared to innovate;
- always developing ways to teach;
- commitment to professional conduct;
- advocate of learner as peripheral participant (see Lave & Wenger; Chapter 1[5]).

Launer[6] summarized the role as 'intelligent conversation with a colleague about a case or issue'.

Activity 7.2

Encouraging a good educational environment

Thinking back to why adults want to learn is a good place to start:

- What is their personal motivation? Are the junior doctors interested and eager to learn (internal motivation) or do they want to learn simply to pass an exam (external motivation)?
- Is the topic meaningful? Is the topic relevant to junior doctors' current work or future plans? Have you made it clear why it is important?
- Is the ward round experience focused? Is learning linked to the work junior doctors are doing and based on the care they are giving patients?
- Appropriate level of knowledge. Is learning pitched at the correct level for junior doctors' stage of training?
- Are there clear learning outcomes? Have you articulated these for the session/attachment/year so that everyone knows where you are heading?
- Is there active involvement? Do junior doctors have the opportunity to be actively involved in the learning process, to influence the outcomes and process?

- Is there regular feedback? Do junior doctors know how well they are doing? Have you told them what they are doing well, as well as what areas could be improved?
- Is there time for reflection? Have you given junior doctors time and encouragement to reflect on the subject and their performance?
  What should be avoided is the following:[11]

  "Unfortunately, many clinical teaching sessions still involve the doctor lecturing on their pet topic in the ward seminar room with not a patient in sight."

Chapter 8 **E-learning**

8.1 Learning outcomes

By the end of this chapter you will be able to demonstrate an understanding of:
- the advantages and challenges for e-learning;
- how to facilitate group online discussions;
- how to develop an e-learning module.

8.2 Introduction

E-learning has very simple roots: lectures in PowerPoint were placed on the web and the result was called e-learning. The inevitable outcome was that some of the worst features of the conventional lecture (such as a lack of interactivity) were transplanted onto the computer screen.

The students we teach today are 'children of the PlayStation generation'. Marc Prensky[1] coined the phrase 'digital natives and digital immigrants' to emphasize the divide between the author's generation and the new generations of students who have been immersed in online media since birth: Accordingly, they make higher demands on systems and structures.

Many of the medical colleges have developed and continue to develop virtual learning environments by asking clinicians to provide material. Clinical medics have typically tried to make sure that the factual content is accurate and relevant, but have not necessarily given much consideration to the specific requirements and opportunities of online media. This situation is slowly being addressed, and more recent online environments are engaging learners in a more effective and dynamic way. We will go on to look at how this is done.

How to Teach Continuing Medical Education. By Mike Davis and Kirsty Forrest. Published 2008 by Blackwell Publishing. ISBN: 978-1-4051-5398-0

8.3 E-learning – advantages and challenges

E-learning has many advantages for the learner, but perhaps the most significant is encapsulated in the phrase 'anytime, anyplace'. Material can be revisited, perused at varying speeds and include self-assessments. For the teacher, there is the ability to provide teaching to large groups over a wide geographical area. However, it is wrong to think that e-learning is cost free, as the design, delivery and maintenance of e-learning courses will need initial capital and further resources. Some of the benefits and related challenges of e-learning are summarized in Table 8.1.

Table 8.1 Benefits and challenges of e-learning.

Benefits	Challenges
Convenience of time and place	Increased time on task and a tendency to access the site at all hours of the day
Ability to repeat parts of the course and do at own pace	Feelings of information overload
Increased access to databases and a wealth of online resources	Technical frustrations because of the steep learning curve for any new platform, access problems, password difficulties
A written discussion aids the process of critical reflection	The written discussion sometimes inhibits learners who prefer the spoken word and can have greater potential for misunderstandings
Students can have ready access to a tutor or facilitator	Students expect immediate responses from tutor. Disjointed nature of conversation because of time delay can be frustrating
Cost effective because of reduction in travel, hotels, time away from work	The development costs can be high

Some of the challenges appear too difficult to overcome. For example, take skills teaching. Conventionally, the preferred method of teaching skills is the four-stage approach – all four stages taking place in a single session. However, as explored in Chapter 5, an online approach to skills teaching might consist of video clips of stages 1 and 2 followed by reinforcement and practice in a face-to-face session. An advantage of this would be that the video could include close-up shots of the skill, interspersed with clinical information or contexts, diagrams and photographs. Furthermore, online learners can play the video as many times as they want, both before and after a face-to-face session.

8.4 Communities of practice

E-learning can be a social way of learning. There are chat rooms where groups can discuss personal as well as work-related topics. There can be more formal discussions around clinical topics, either synchronous or asynchronous. The key characteristics of these discussions are shown in Table 8.2.

The asynchronous discussion has a place in the lives of busy clinicians who find it difficult to make arrangements for face-to-face meetings, teleconferences or online synchronous conferences.

Blended learning

As is evident from Table 8.2, face-to-face discussions are the hardest to organize but are a helpful component of an online course. This type of teaching, involving both synchronous and asynchronous activity, is called blended learning.

Students are most likely to succeed in a distance learning program if:

• they are self-motivated and good at setting and meeting their own deadlines;
• they use email frequently and find it a satisfactory way to communicate;
• they enjoy spending time by themselves at their computer.

Obviously, this is not all learners; e-learning will not appeal to those who need face-to-face contact with teachers or fellow learners. Therefore, using a blended approach to teaching will help to include all learners. A blended approach gives the opportunity to develop good group dynamics (i.e. a group that can function), with a clear sense of purpose, secure boundaries and the ability to manage conflict and disagreement. This is particularly important and much harder to achieve online when participants find it difficult to

Table 8.2 Forms of interaction/discussion.

	Same time	Different time
Same place	Face-to-face meeting. This could be at the beginning of a training module as a general introduction – say, in computer cluster to take you through the technical aspects of the course	Smaller groups – could get together at a computer cluster and feed back to the larger group online
Different place	Synchronous online discussion. Usually at a set time arranged in the course	Asynchronous discussion – the same as having an email conversation

sense who they are writing to. Some of the difficulties associated with online communication were identified by Davis in an online article.[2]

Online educational environments can therefore sometimes supplement rather than replace face-to-face activity. However, they can be useful for the transference of knowledge-based content and for discussions about case studies.

Discussion groups in practice – an example

The following is an example for anaesthetic registrars in one training region. Case presentations are placed online every 8–10 days and all trainees are expected to participate in the discussion over that time. The discussion is held in password-protected fora which the trainees are invited to sign into.

A topic begins with limited information:

> How would you anaesthetize a 30-year-old for a k-wiring of a fractured forearm?

Trainees post their anaesthetic plan (there is emphasis on the fact there is no right or wrong answer). More information is then posted:

> The patient has an active chest infection.

The trainees then say how and why their plans would change. This type of teaching can explore decision-making practices of the trainee. Discussion continues between trainees and facilitators. A tutorial is held at the end of each case scenario where nominated trainees present the themes from the discussions and a summary of the relevant literature. Any misconceptions that may have surfaced during the online discussion can be tackled at this time.

8.5 E-moderating

Facilitating an online discussion is similar in certain ways to facilitating a face-to-face open discussion. There are behaviours that encourage learning and others that do not. They are very similar to the behaviours of people within groups discussed in Chapter 4. For example, lack of interest and socializing, ignoring the process and being passive can be online behaviours that would have an effect on the group dynamics. Facilitators have to be aware when these behaviours arise and prevent them from becoming the norm. However, there are some differences to facilitating online groups and these have been summarized by Gilly Salmon[3] and termed e-moderating.

The five-step process for e-moderating is summarized below.

Step 1. Access and motivation

Students are led through the initial stages of making their first links to the course site and associated materials. (Some students may need help with the 'technical'/IT skills required for such connections.) It is vital that at this stage the students are supported and encouraged to participate – they should feel welcomed and encouraged. This stage will end when students have successfully undertaken a sample of typical e-learning tasks such as posting a message in a discussion group or completing a simple assessment.

Step 2. Online socialization

Students begin to interact socially with others in the (online) class, because they have become familiar with the communication tools and are adopting the particular 'culture' that such tools demand. This should result in a sense of group identity. Not all students will develop at the same rate; some will 'lurk' in the background. This is normal for online group activity but such students should be gently drawn into online discussions and activities – otherwise they are in danger of 'dropping out'. Similarly, students who are 'up front' and tend to dominate group discussions should be gently reminded of the need to let others have their say. This may have to be done in a private email or by telephone.

Step 3. Information exchange

Students become actively involved with course content and activity, beginning to exchange information and views with others in the class. They develop personal approaches to dealing with the information and messages that end in their 'inbox'; such approaches may need to be encouraged by tutors alongside the provision of stimulation and motivation in the use of support materials and guidance on information sharing.

Step 4. Knowledge construction

At stage 4, students start to actively construct knowledge rather than simply receive and transfer information. They do this by sharing personal knowledge and opinions, critiquing and building on course content and on one another's contributions to course discussions, often around problem or project-based topics. The role of the tutor becomes one of facilitator and moderator of these discussions – stimulating contribution, summarizing progress and weaving together different threads.

Step 5. Development

Finally, students become responsible for their own learning within this new online medium. Students are motivated by their own personal interest and experience to explore the topic area being studied. Tutors move from facilitating discussions to supporting and responding to participants as they define and lead their own discussions.

8.6 How to design an e-learning module

Needs analysis

E-learning is suitable for many types of teaching interventions, but is particularly good where gaining knowledge is the key. When embarking on the development of e-learning material, the first question that needs to be answered is: 'Is e-learning the right solution?' In order to answer this question, the following questions will also need to be considered:

- What is expected of the online course?
- Will it replace or supplement existing teaching?
- Is an online course the best choice?
- What will the costs be and who will maintain and update the course?
- Who will finally approve the course? What are his/her expectations?
   This needs analysis should also include a user analysis:
- Who are the target students?
- Will they be able to access the course site and perform all the necessary interactions?
- How will students benefit from the online course?
- How can students progress be evaluated?

   These are the ideal characteristics that a teacher needs to develop e-learning materials:

- knowledge of adult learning theory.
- instructional design competence and knowledge of different e-learning solutions;
- skills to use the e-learning development software tool;
- an awareness of basic graphic design principles;
- the skills to manipulate images in a graphic design software tool.

   However, some clinicians are too busy to become proficient in the use of authoring tools such as Dreamweaver. Often, Internet designers will do the authoring for you; however, when writing the material bearing in mind the way it will be viewed and presented is vital. Also, the basics for all education should not be lost: having educational goals, providing 'the learning', assessing lessons learned and providing feedback.

Educational goals

Clearly define the objectives of the course. Keep it practical and relevant to real world situations. Give students guidelines by which to evaluate their performance. Build accurate expectations from the course:

- What are the educational goals?
- How will these goals be accomplished?

- Which goals will possibly not be accomplished and how can we compensate for them?
- What approaches could be used to achieve a given goal?

Design considerations

Often, you will be adapting material you already have – previous lectures or book chapters. Even this material may have to be rewritten for course content on the web. Keep the language simple and friendly, especially if there is no teacher contact to provide the human touch you will need to present the content in a non-threatening way. Incorporate motivational elements such as certificates on completion and discussion boards for interaction with other students. Prepare a flow chart or story board showing how the course progresses from start to finish. The pages containing the course material should be organized in a way that makes navigation easy and simple (Fig. 8.1).

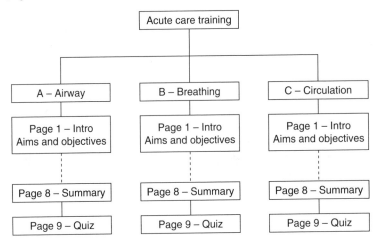

Figure 8.1 An example of flow chart.

The material will need to be 'chunked'; there is a temptation to put too much information in each unit. Think about when you look at a computer screen and what you would like to see:

- Allow for easy scanning because a high percentage of web users read that way.
- Use plenty of sub-headings and ensure that the main points are emphasized visually.
- Use pictures, graphs or tables where they would aid learning.

- Provide links for further information to journal articles or other websites that could be of interest to the student.
- Each page should be able to be visualized on one screen shot (i.e. the learner should not have to scroll down the page).
- Normal design and presentation styles apply as for using PowerPoint, keep the font readable and do not overuse colour.

In addition, the use of video and audio clips can add to the richness and complexity of the material. As an example, a videoed case conference or examination can add considerably to the text.

Publication

What options are there for actually publishing your e-learning material (i.e. making it accessible online)? You all are probably too aware that there are more and more possibilities for publishing your material every year. To help you narrow down the choice, think about your answers to the following questions.

Do you have someone at your university or institution who can look after the mechanics of getting the material online for you? This will often be the best option, as they will be experienced with the systems in use at your institution, but of course you may have to compete with others for their time, and you have less control over the final outcome.

Alternatively, are you happy to get your hands 'dirty' and tackle the technical requirements yourself? This may not be as difficult as you think, as the web is increasingly a 'read–write' medium. By doing it yourself you gain ultimate control over what appears online (as well as ultimate responsibility for maintaining it).

There is a range of options of increasing sophistication.

Plain HTML

HTML itself is not the hardest thing to write using a decent editor, or you can use a WYSIWYG (what you see is what you get!) tool such as Dreamweaver or iWeb to create attractively presented pages.

Content management system

Your institution probably offers some facility for creating and publishing personal content, and if it does not, there are plenty of other places that do. A blog (or web log) is just a content management system (CMS) that presents your content in the form of a journal and, depending on your requirements, this may be all you need to present your thoughts (e.g. CMSs: Google Pages (pages.google.com), blogger.com, wordpress.com).

Learning Management System

A learning management system (LMS) is a specific type of CMS with extra functionality to support the sort of things that learners and tutors need (e.g. the in-house LMS at Leeds University supports these features):

- lecture presentations, video, images, lecture handouts and other teaching support materials;
- electronic discussion groups;
- quizzes and surveys;
- electronic submission of assignments via 'pigeonhole' area;
- web and library resources (e.g. course relevant websites, full text journal article databases, subject resources);
- log book of learning reflections and student personal development.

You do not need to use all these features to make it worth your while using an LMS. Examples of current LMSs that might be available to you include moodle, dokeos, bodington and sakai. All of these are available as free downloads, so your institution may be able to offer these to you if you ask for them.

Testing

Design your test questions keeping the course objectives in mind. It is often easier to think of these questions while you develop the material. The idea is to evaluate the student's learning and provide constructive feedback where necessary. Vague and confusing questions should be avoided. Predeveloped quiz scripts can be installed, programmed with the correct answers and feedback. Multiple choice and true/false questions are the most popular.

You will have to prepare:

- test/question;
- possible answer choices;
- correct answer + feedback;
- wrong answer + feedback.

Layout and interface design

Navigation should be simple and intuitive. The student needs to be oriented about where he/she is within the course. A uniform look and feel can be developed for the entire course. This includes colours, background and graphics.

Usability testing

The module should then be piloted on students, their reactions noted and suitable changes made. You may realize that the interface is not as intuitive as you thought or that the student expected something else entirely when they clicked on a certain button. Any frustration in getting to a certain required piece of information should also be noted and action taken accordingly.

Once the interface prototype is tested and finalized, a template can be created. Using the flow chart for reference, all the pages can be created with a blank space for the content. All these pages can be linked and the navigation tested for functionality.

Online testing and evaluation

Once your course goes online, you will find that some things that worked fine on your local computer do not work as well from a remote server.

- Your material may contain direct links to files (e.g. images, media) that are only present on your own computer.
- There will inevitably be some technical differences with the remote server, these can sometimes cause problems (e.g. with the text encoding of the files).
- Bandwidth constraints can slow down or even truncate the downloading of pages and graphics.
- Whenever possible, test or preview the material from a different computer than you used to create the course (e.g. to ensure that all the images have been uploaded).
- Get someone else to read it through and look for major howlers. It helps if they are using a different computer, browser or operating system. It may also help if they are not too computer literate, as your goal is to make the material as accessible as possible for everybody.

8.7 Conclusions

To provide this best e-learning experience, keep in mind the following points:

- Provide the learner with an introduction to the course which includes key information, how to work through it and how it applies to their practice.
- Ensure the content is structured into meaningful chunks and arranged into a sequence.
- Use a variety of approaches designed to meet the differing needs of learners.
- Pre- and post-assessment tests can be included when appropriate. When using multiple choice questions, make sure they are clear and unambiguous with plausible distracters.
- Introduce feedback that is comprehensive, helpful and, where possible, directly related to the learner's answer.

- Navigation should be simple and clear, allowing the learner to easily navigate around the course and lessons. Consider recording progress automatically.
- Give consideration to the appropriate use of animation, audio and video that enhance the learning experience but should not be used gratuitously.

The web is becoming a well-used forum for the delivery of CME. How best to develop and deliver this material are important questions for clinical teachers.

References

1 Prensky M. Digital natives, digital immigrants. *On the Horizon* 2001;9(5). NCB University Press.

2 Davis M. Fragmented by technologies: A community in cybserpace. *Interpersonal Computing and Technology* 1997;**5**:1–2,7–18.

3 Salmon G. *E-moderating: The Key to Teaching and Learning Online* (2nd edn). 2004. Taylor and Francis, London.

Chapter 9 **Annotated bibliography**

Bloom BS. *Taxonomy of Educational Objectives, Handbook 1: The Cognitive Domain*. 1956. David McKay, New York.

This, and the books on the affective and psychomotor domains that followed it, had a profound significance on the way in which the structure of educational events was conceived. While resisting attempts to use the taxonomies as a straightjacket, the educator can take advantage of the insights into ways of thinking about knowledge, skills, and attitudes having several dimensions.

Boud D, Cohen R, Walker D. (eds.) *Using Experience for Learning*. 1993. SRHE/Open University Press, Buckingham.

One of a number of important collaborations on the contribution of reflection to adult learning in higher education and professional practice.

Brookfield S. *Becoming a Critically Reflective Teacher*. 1995. Jossey-Bass, San Francisco.

This is a powerful account of some of the sociopsychological issues associated with being a teacher. As King and Hibbison say in their review:

> In order to be successful in becoming critically reflective, Brookfield asserts that the teacher must use four critically reflective lenses:
> - the teacher's unique autobiography as a teacher and learner, using personal self-reflection and collecting the insights and meanings for teaching;
> - making an assessment of one's self through the students' lens by seeking their input and seeing classrooms and learning from their perspectives;

How to Teach Continuing Medical Education. By Mike Davis and Kirsty Forrest. Published 2008 by Blackwell Publishing. ISBN: 978-1-4051-5398-0

- by peer review of teaching from a colleague's experiences, observations and feedback;
- by frequently referring to the theoretical literature that may provide an alternative interpretive framework for a situation.

One reason offered by Brookfield for relying on the theoretical literature was because 'it becomes a psychological and political survival necessity through which teachers come to understand the link between their private troubles and broader political processes'.

The implications of critical reflection on teaching are many: (1) it leads to the realization that teaching and curricula are grounded in ideology; (2) it helps teachers discover how to minimize their risk of doing damage to themselves, or at least, keeping it to a minimum; (3) it allows one to see himself or herself as constantly evolving and growing; (4) it allows teachers to create connections between educational processes, students' experiences of learning and what they feel important concerns in their lives; (5) it contributes to the creation of more democratic learning environments because as a result of critical reflection, teachers are able to create conditions where all voices can speak and be heard in the classroom and where educational processes are genuinely open to negotiation and (6) finally, teachers come into their own and discover their authentic voices.

(King R, Hibbison P. The importance of critical reflection in college teaching: Two reviews of Stephen Brookfield's book, *Becoming a Critically Reflective Teacher. Inquiry* 2000; **5**:2.)

Bullock I, Davis M, Lockey A, Mackway-Jones K. (eds.) *Pocket Guide to Teaching for Medical Instructors* (2nd edn). 2008. Blackwell, Oxford.

An updated version of the extremely popular first edition aimed predominantly, but not exclusively, at instructors working on Advanced Life Support Group (ALSG) and Resuscitation Council (RC) (UK) resuscitation courses.

Dent J, Harden R. (eds.) *A Practical Guide for Medical Teachers* (2nd edn.) 2005. Churchill Livingstone, Edinburgh.

A substantial book divided into seven sections: curriculum; learning situations; educational strategies; tools/aids; curriculum themes; assessment and students and staff. As the editors write in their preface:

It is the purpose of this book to address [the] task [of] bridging the gap between theoretical aspects of medical education and its attendant jargon, and the practical delivery of enthusiastic teaching.

The book is an attempt to help clinicians especially, and other health care teachers in general, in their understanding of contemporary educational principles and to provide practical help for them in the delivery of the variety of teaching situations which characterize the present day curricula.

Dewey J. *How We Think: A Restatement of the Relation of Reflective Thinking to the Educative Process* (revised edn.). 1933. DC Heath, Boston.

Dewey laid the foundations for explorations of the significance of collaborative learning; the nature and potential of experience; and reflective practice. His books made a significant contribution to the thinking of authors such as David Boud (on reflection), David Kolb (learning from experience), and Schön (the reflective practitioner). A new edition of this work was published in 2007.

Knowles MS. *The Adult Learner: A Neglected Species* (4th edn.). 1990. Gulf Publishing, Houston.

A seminal work on adult learning, this book surveys adult learning theories and explores further his notion of andragogy which has been described as 'the art of helping adults learn' as opposed to pedagogy, 'the science or art of teaching'.

Kolb D. *Experiential Learning: Experiences as the Source of Learning and Development.* 1984. Prentice-Hall, Englewood Cliffs.

An exploration of the significance of learning from experience and what is required to develop the capacity to do so. Further work with Fry (Kolb D, Fry R. Toward an applied theory of experiential learning. In Cooper C. (ed.) *Theories of Group Process.* 1975. John Wiley, London) created the learning styles inventory.

While aspects of Kolb's work has been criticized for its apparent inattention to detail, it still makes a valuable contribution to understanding of what is required if we are to learn from experience.

Lave J, Wenger E. *Situated Learning: Legitimate Peripheral Participation.* 1991. University of Cambridge, Cambridge.

Lave and Wenger's book was in response to the notion that learning 'has a beginning and an end; that it is best separated from the rest of our activities; and that it is the result of teaching' (Wenger E. Communities of practice: learning as a social system.*Systems Thinker* 1998. http://www.co-i-l.com/coil/knowledge-garden/cop/lss.shtml accessed on 25 October 2007.)

Lave and Wenger use observations of people learning in different social contexts from midwives, to tailors, to members of Alcoholics Anonymous as the basis of their theory of the community of practice. Learning is seen as a social phenomenon, rather than something that goes on only in the head of an individual learner. Clearly, learning when viewed in this way is not simply facts and their application, but a way of thinking about self and others functioning in a shared community.

Lewin, K. (1951) *Field theory in social science; selected theoretical papers*, pp. 162. D. Cartwright (ed.). New York: Harper & Row.

Almost all of Kurt Lewin's publications appeared after his death in editions edited by his graduate students, many of whom became major contributors to our understanding of adult learning, particularly in groups. He is also credited with creating the idea of 'action research', described as:

> A form of self-reflective enquiry undertaken by participants in social situations in order to improve the rationality and justice of their own practices, their understanding of these practices, and the situations in which the practices are carried out.' (Carr W, Kemmis S. *Becoming Critical: Education, Knowledge and Action Research*. 1986. Falmer, Lewes).

More recent collection of Lewin's work can be found in Gold M. *The Complete Social Scientist*. 1999. APA Books, Washington.

Maslow, A. A theory of human motivation. *Psychological Review* 1943; **50**:370–396. [http://psychclassics.yorku.ca/Maslow/motivation.htm accessed in June 2001]

By visiting this site, you will be able to see the original article, which has been a major contributor to thinking about motivation and how that impacts on learning. Maslow's theories have some critics, the most unusual one being based on his research methodology.

Mezirow J, *et al.* (eds.) *Fostering Critical Reflection in Adulthood*. 1990. Jossey-Bass, San Francisco.

According to Mezirow, the role of the adult educator is to:
• help the learner focus on and examine the assumptions that underlie their beliefs, feelings and actions;
• assess the consequences of these assumptions;
• identify and explore alternative sets of assumptions;
• test the validity of assumptions through effective participation in reflective dialogue.

Transformative learning involves:
• becoming more reflective and critical;

- being more open to the perspectives of others;
- being less defensive and more accepting of new ideas.

Mezirow states that as transformative educators, we 'may help others, and perhaps ourselves, move toward a fuller and more dependable understanding of the meaning of our mutual experience'.

Newble D, Cannon R. *A Handbook for Medical Teachers* (4th edn.). 2001. Kluwer Academic, Dordrecht.

Probably the first book aimed at medical educators when it first appeared over 25 years ago and now in its fourth edition and still well regarded.

Schön D. *The Reflective Practitioner: How Professionals Think in Action.* 1983. Basic Books, New York.

Among Schön's concerns was that university education did not necessarily relate to the day-to-day practices of the expert practitioner. In a review of Schon's contribution to design education, Waks wrote:

> The crisis of the professions arises because real-life problems do not present themselves neatly as cases to which scientific generalizations apply. So this epistemology of technical rationality eventually leads to a dilemma of *rigor vs. relevance.* Professional practitioners find themselves pursuing either arcane technical studies more or less inapplicable to the 'swamps' of real-life practice, or significant real-life problems which call for approaches not deemed 'rational' or 'scientific' when judged by the standards of university professional schools. Practicum instructors are caught in the dilemma of having to teach real-life practice when they are supposed to be teaching something else, applied science. (Waks L. Donald Schön's philosophy of design and design education. *International Journal of Technology and Design Education* 2001;**11**:37–51.

Schön's target behaviour for professionals is the capacity to reflect-in-action, rather than reflect-on-action. However, the capacity to engage in the latter may be a prerequisite of the former.

Those interested in continuing medical education should consider membership of:

Association of Medical Education in Europe (AMEE) which publishes *Medical Teacher* 12 times a year and holds an annual conference. See http://www.amee.org

Association for the Study of Medical Education (ASME) which publishes *Medical Education* 12 times a year and also holds an annual conference. See www.asme.org.uk

Academy of Medical Educators has recently come into existence and this will be offering membership and fellowship from early in 2008. See www.medicaleducators.org.

Index